LIVING A LIFE OF VITALITY

LIVING A LIFE OF VITALITY

VITALITY

A Mind, Body, and Spirit Approach

GRETCHEN LEE ADAMS

Editing by Deborah Ager; Copyediting by Heather Trimm

Front cover photo of Maria and Brett Beveridge by Gretchen Lee Adams, used with permission

Back cover image by Amandamatildaphotography.com

Cover and book design by Beehive Book Design

*To my family who always support me in
whatever crazy endeavor I conjure up.*

CONTENTS

LIVING A LIFE OF VITALITY

INTRODUCTION

Autoimmune disease: when the body attacks and damages its own tissues.

MORE THAN FIVE YEARS AGO, I thought I knew myself well, including my strengths and weaknesses, and I thought I knew what my future looked like. An autoimmune diagnosis turned my world upside down and sent me reeling to various doctors and specialists only to find few answers and no cures. I was now a member of a "special" group of over 50 million people, those with autoimmune disease. There are between 80 and 100 types of autoimmune disease all based on the same principles: your immune system for unknown reasons attacks itself.

At age 60, after a lifetime blessed with good health, I had my first "incident." I lost 40% of my hair. I wasn't prepared to have a medical issue arise, especially a mystery one. I cried in the shower when my hair came out in handfuls, and I fully experienced trauma associated with losing my hair without knowing why. Eventually, my hair regrew but not without a lot of heartache and struggle.

In the midst of that first incident, I visited my horrified hair stylist, who sent me to her internist. I was in Florida at the time. Massive blood tests began. Did I have cancer? Did I have something else that would impact my long-term health? I worried. The blood work results returned as all normal and offered no reasons to explain the hair loss. Only a random guess of mine pinpointed what we thought to be the cause: a brief and limited use of an estrogen cream, which buried "hair loss possible" deep in the list of side effects. Thankfully, the bald patches that appeared on my head could be hidden with styling. In my mind, it was just a matter of time for the hair to grow back. It never entered my mind I would lose my hair more than once.

Nearly a year later, my hair started falling out again. This time, I visited my regular doctor back home in Colorado. Since the hair loss was still in the early stages, there wasn't much to see—no visible thinning of my hair or bald patches—so my doctor looked at me with disbelief, clearly re-evaluating what kind of patient I was. But I *knew* what was happening. One look at the heap of hair in my bathroom sink told me everything. I insisted on receiving blood tests with an emphasis on the thyroid, because thyroid issues run in my family. The bloodwork showed normal results again, but this time I had no medication or estrogen cream to point a finger at as I had before. I was baffled. Meanwhile, my doctor thought I was a kook, and hair continued to fall out like silent snowflakes from the sky. My husband and I traveled to our Florida home with no answers.

Next, I visited my dermatologist, who I normally visited only once a year for a skin checkup. She diagnosed me with alopecia areata and finally put a name to this condition. Alopecia is an autoimmune disease in which the body attacks its own hair follicles. As with all autoimmune diseases, there's no cure. The dermatologist suggested trying steroids to put it into remission. After a lifetime of medication avoidance, and in a current state of panic, I agreed to receive a shot right then and there. I'd later receive a series of weekly shots. Steroids have a host of side effects and are controversial. My concerned family intervened and encouraged me to seek out an alternative doctor as a safer option. A good friend recommended a doctor, and my path took another turn.

Dr. John Patton, my new alternative doctor, is a board-certified Doctor of Acupuncture and Oriental Medicine (DAOM), and a licensed psychotherapist and mental health counselor with more than 50 years of experience practicing in the healthcare industry. After intense questioning about seemingly everything I had ever said, done, or put in my mouth, he wanted me to overhaul my diet, learn daily meditation, avoid stressful situations (including violent movies and books), start weekly acupuncture treatments and counseling sessions, and have adrenal testing. After that first session, I felt shell shocked and thrust into an unknown world: the world of alternative medicine.

My adrenal test results showed such extreme adrenal fatigue that it alarmed the lab. I was immediately placed on a program of adrenal supplements. Dr. Patton theorized that my lifetime way of dealing with life's stresses no longer worked well for me and that, combined with aging, caused my immune system to go haywire. Boom. An autoimmune disease.

I lost 40% of my hair again before it stopped. The cycle of slow and uneven regrowth started again. A few months passed, and I felt invigorated by my new practices of acupuncture and meditation. An adrenal re-test showed I was back in the "normal" range. While there were no definitive answers as to why my autoimmune issues had started, I felt all was under control. But that feeling would not last long.

I awoke one morning to find hair all over my pillow. My heart sank. This third hair loss event, occurring 15 months after the second event, was instant and fierce. I lost 50% of my hair in two weeks. Over the next six weeks, I lost 100% of the hair over my entire body, including my eyebrows, eyelashes, legs, arms, ears, and nose. We had no idea why it happened. I was in a good place mentally and physically, and blood test results showed nothing. I was forced to dive into a world I knew nothing about: the world of wigs. Life had to continue. While I had been knocked down, I came back up fighting.

While I adjusted to life with wigs, I started researching everything I could about autoimmune disease and health in the US. Some interesting facts emerged. My research turned up an alarming increase in certain kinds of disorders—hypertension, diabetes, coronary arterial disease, and autoimmune diseases—in the US. In fact, the rate of escalating autoimmune diseases is high in most developed countries in the world and show no signs of slowing. Only theories from experts suggest why.

My growing list of doctors, which now included a specialist in alopecia, did not have answers for me either. The most plausible explanation I found was a theory held by a number of medical experts. The theory proposes that we begin life with what is essentially a "bucket," or limit, to what our individual immune system can tolerate with regard to toxicity. We are all exposed to a myriad of toxic substances through the air, what we drink and eat, and what we come into contact with through the skin. When the amount of toxicity exceeds the capacity of the "bucket," the immune system becomes over challenged. As a result, autoimmune response strikes, and disorders and disease appear. The amount of toxicity that an immune system can handle is unique to each individual, and no way currently exists to predetermine that limit.

If correct, the theory would suggest my immune system hit capacity with the original hair event. That would mean I had to do everything possible to strengthen and repair my immune system and make any changes that could hopefully stave off future attacks. Effective medications to eliminate symptoms for my particular autoimmune disease do not exist. Even if medication existed, I would have to weigh the consequences of potentially harmful side effects against avoiding future hair loss. Non-drug treatments are my preference because many drugs prescribed today come with serious side effects.

Although I consider us an over-prescribed nation here in the US, I found a growing intersection between Western traditional medicine and Eastern medicine and the ways practitioners offered holistic alternatives for patients. I tell my friends now to seek doctors specializing in functional or integrative medicine, because both disciplines work to treat the whole person and find root causes to disorders and diseases. Realizing that mind, body, and spirit are all inescapably intertwined, I felt forced to re-examine my purpose and goals in life along with my health and habits. This book comes from my search. Anyone can make changes to improve their general health, strengthen their immune systems, and have a stronger body and mind to withstand the ravages of illness.

This book is my experience and what I learned through research. I have made every effort to publish accurate information. Given that science constantly evolves, there may be inaccuracies. It is not intended to be a substitute for professional medical advice.

Before you dismiss autoimmune disease as having nothing to do with you, please know that it can appear suddenly and without warning. Diseases you are familiar with have a basis in autoimmune disorders. The list continues to grow with newly discovered ones. Many more of us are at risk for developing an autoimmune disease than we realize. I had no prior health issues that would have alerted me of the trouble to come.

According to the American Autoimmune Related Diseases Association (AARDA), there are 80-100 autoimmune diseases that affect more than 50 million people, including:

- Alopecia Areata
- Lupus
- Rheumatoid arthritis
- Inflammatory bowel disease (IBD)
- Multiple Sclerosis (MS)
- Psoriasis
- Guillain-Barre syndrome
- Type 1 Diabetes
- Vasculitis
- Myasthenia gravis
- Graves' disease (hyperthyroidism)
- Hashimoto's thyroiditis (hypothyroidism)
- Celiac disease
- Interstitial cystitis (IC)
- Restless leg syndrome (RLS)
- Ulcerative colitis (UC)

For a complete list, visit aarda.org.

Given the severity of many autoimmune diseases, I consider myself lucky. Mine doesn't have the debilitating symptoms that others do, and I haven't developed another autoimmune disease, which can occur once you have developed a first one. The main symptom for alopecia is hair loss, which manifests in varying degrees—alopecia areata, which is partial hair loss (generally limited to the head) to the most severe alopecia universalis (total hair loss over the body). Although it's not physically debilitating, hair loss carries emotional trauma and social stigma with it, especially for women. Our attachment to our physical selves and modern society's emphasis on the outwardly physical rather than the internal puts us in that realm in the first place.

Some people are born with health issues, and others develop health issues early in life. Then, there are the rest of us. We may have followed a strict health regimen for years or ignored the current health advice altogether. Regardless, at some point we may find ourselves at a crossroads. Maybe we develop a disorder or a more serious disease, or we might have difficulty healing from an injury which requires a doctor, surgery and/or drug intervention. As we get older, our immune system—a complex network of cells, tissues, and organs—loses its ability to work as well as it did in our younger years. Scientists do not fully understand why, but this puts people at a higher risk of becoming ill.

What happened to me is a warning that we're all running a much higher risk than we realize of developing disorders and diseases. The latest statistics from the CDC (Centers for Disease Control) show we have more health issues than ten years ago even though we have a longer life expectancy than previous generations. Diabetes, obesity, and hypertension, to name a few, plague our generation. Diseases, such as coronary artery disease, have a cause and effect that doctors say can be directly attributed to our unhealthy diets and lack of exercise. While cancer deaths continue to decrease due to better treatments, we see an increase in the incidence of some types of cancer in both adults and children. Recent large-scale studies show alarming changes in human conditions, such as dramatically lowered male fertility and serious sudden onset adult food allergies. Scientists believe all of these happen at a rate that is too high and rapid to be attributed solely to genetic changes. They surmise the cause to be environmental, but we don't have complete answers yet.

On the positive front, new scientific and medical research is already leading to discoveries that bring us ever closer to curing major diseases. A lot of this is based on the overriding premise that the human body has an astounding ability to heal itself. These life-changing possibilities indicate that we have enormous potential to expand our brain power, heal ourselves, and live long vibrant lives. Some of these are new discoveries using the latest modern technology, and some are drawing upon ancient knowledge passed on by indigenous peoples, which recent studies have given newfound validity. Bottom line: the human body has untapped capabilities that are only just now being discovered.

A word of caution: When it comes to deciphering between new verified scientific medical discoveries and companies attempting to sell their unproven products to the public, no "fix it" or "anti-aging" pill has been proven to work nor has the FDA approved any. Be wary of any group or company who touts themselves as having the magic solution. What appears to be a more viable approach to good health and vibrant long life includes overhauling diet and exercise routines, managing stress, incorporating nature in our activities, and eliminating as many toxins from our environment as possible. Sigh, a magic pill *would* be much easier.

We can find a million diets and exercise programs, so how do we know which to choose? While this is not a diet and exercise book, those two subjects rank high on the priority list in the overall scheme of taking care of ourselves. I dedicate a chapter to each. I break down what is consistent over many decades of medical research—with "consistent" being the key word. The sheer magnitude of the studies makes it easier to see patterns among all types of people regarding diet and exercise.

However, as it turns out, **exercise and diet are only part of the solution**. If we add taking care of our brains, managing modern day stress, finding a purpose in our lives, and locating ways to eliminate some of the toxicity in our immediate environment, we will be miles ahead of the ultimate goal: a long life lived with vitality. Although these changes probably sound overwhelming, a lot of the process involves making small changes that add up to a big impact over time.

What could be causing all the increased health issues? Experts maintain various theories, but there is consistent alarm over the high rate of obesity and lack of exercise combined with concern over toxicity in our air, water, food and products we use on and in our bodies and in our environments.

Obesity sets the body up for a multitude of disorders and diseases that can shorten a person's lifespan. An unhealthy diet and a sedentary lifestyle are believed to be major contributors to the increasing obesity rate in this country. Regular physical exercise reduces your risk of disease, increases mental well-being, helps you stay in good shape to avoid injury, safely perform work tasks and leisure activities, and can lengthen your lifespan. Startling statistics from the CDC indicate only 22.9% of adults (18-64) exercise regularly in the US[1]. While we are bombarded by marketing messages for every form of diet and exercise, and gyms open on every corner, many only *talk* about exercise and healthy eating. Billions of dollars are spent on special diets, exercise equipment, and gym memberships. It seems the majority of people briefly try the products out and discard them.

The US average diet is full of processed and highly salted and sugared foods. Vegetables and fruits are eaten in lower quantities than what's recommended for good health. Fast food purveyors win over the taste buds of the American public with heavily processed foods of all types. While in recent years they have added healthier options and now provide fat, sodium, sugar, and calorie content to their menu boards, the discipline it requires to order

---

1 "National Health Statistics Reports, Number 112, June 28, 2018-CDC." Accessed May 4, 2019. https://www.cdc.gov/nchs/data/nhsr/nhsr112.pdf.

the healthier foods proves difficult for most of us. For me, it's a dangerous option, because I love the taste of it. As a result, I stay away from it all as much as possible.

As I continued my research on how to live a healthy life, "toxicity" came up repeatedly.

Definition of toxic: poisonous.

Scientists tell us there is no longer 100% pure air or water on this planet. Even in the most inaccessible places, traces of chemical substances can be found in people's blood and urine. Newborn babies are born with minute traces of foreign substances. Our food sources have come under increasing scrutiny due to an ever-growing concern over what chemicals are being used for crops and in feed for meat sources and how they impact our health. Not to be excluded are the products that we use on our bodies and in our living environment. We are surrounded by chemicals every day – around 80,000, according to the EPA.[2] Some scientists insist the minuscule amounts present in most people create little, if any, health risk while others adamantly state the continually increasing amount of foreign substances *does* put our health at risk.

I thought I knew what products to buy or avoid, but it became apparent early in my research that I was lacking a lot of knowledge. Unfortunately, government supervision

2   "It could take centuries for EPA to test all the unregulated chemicals ...." Accessed May 4, 2019. https://www.pbs.org/newshour/science/it-could-take-centuries-for-epa-to-test-all-the-unregulated-chemicals-under-a-new-landmark-bill.

or testing to oversee the escalating chemical output falls short. FDA processes are slow, and EPA testing is underfunded. This means we have to take control of our own health and acquire enough information to make informed decisions. The realization that I couldn't be confident our government was doing everything needed to ensure what we surround ourselves with was safe sobered me.

We can all incorporate, small, easily accomplished changes that scientists say can make a huge difference in our health and longevity. A priority for me was to make changes that would help strengthen and balance my immune system.

For me—and I think for all of us—this means we need accurate information to take action. Scientists insist our bodies are made to last much longer than the current age predictions: a 120 years or more.[3] These predictions are based, in part, on the current advances in biomedical technology and research into ways that the body's natural repair pathways can be accessed. We are living right in the middle of an explosive era of medical advances. Those advances move at such a fast pace that results of testing are released without fully understanding the "whys." Since acting on these findings has little, if any, risk and the benefits could be enormous, scientists feel it is important to release the information to the public as soon as possible. If you're like most people, you might find it hard to keep up with the verified information or to know the difference

---

3   "There's no limit to longevity, says study that revives human ...–Nature." Accessed May 4, 2019. https://www.nature.com/articles/ d41586-018-05582-3.

between scams and truth. This new world of "fake" news requires close attention to where we are getting our information. I've attempted to try and disseminate the information out there and use reliable, vetted sources to make some sense of it.

We can take action to help ourselves maintain good health, build up immunity, and avoid the consequences of toxicity. These things apply to everyone and not just my own baby boomer generation. Every chapter discusses easy changes we can make. While using these practices earlier will mean you're better off, it's never too late to start. As we age, it's true that it's harder for our bodies to counteract the negative. However, some encouraging recent studies indicate these practices have beneficial results even for much older people.

Each of these categories contain techniques and information to help in the quest to implement self-care and self-healing, including adjusting our environments to a healthier one. You'll likely see a number of things you're already incorporating in your life plus a list of practices to consider and new developments to keep an eye on.

In the process of researching and writing this book, I was frequently asked by a number of friends and family what information I could give them on a variety of health topics. All the questions and the search for answers ultimately led to this book with the chapter categories that follow.

1. Keep Physically Active
2. Eat a Healthy Balanced Diet
3. Manage Stress
4. Spend Time in Nature
5. Take Care of Your Brain
6. Alleviate Toxicity
7. Have a Purpose in Life

Each of these subjects make up part of the puzzle to help you live a long, healthy, and fulfilled life. Although this information can be found from many sources, it takes work and research to find it, so I've pulled it all together in one place for you.

I feel grateful and empowered by all I've learned about taking care of body, mind, and spirit. As there is no current cure for any autoimmune disease, the possibility remains that I could relapse. I try to be prepared for that. As of now, I'm in a three-year remission without illness of any kind—not even a cold. And, yes, my hair did grow back in some fashion but not enough to discard the wigs for now. On the other hand, shaving my legs or underarms is a rare event, which I consider a plus.

The whole experience has made a profound difference in my life and belief systems and even in how I view the world. We are all much more than the physical selves we see. In fact, I now believe the most important parts of us are within. I'm embracing life as never before and believe we can make a difference in our own health mentally, physically, and spiritually. You don't have to rely solely on the next drug, surgery, or doctor to be healthy.

Gretchen Adams
Naples, Florida 2019

KEEP PHYSICALLY ACTIVE

Exercise is activity requiring physical effort, carried out to sustain or improve health and fitness. (Oxfordictionaries.com)

PHYSICAL ACTIVITY IS DEFINED AS any bodily movement produced by skeletal muscles that results in energy expenditure.[4]

My doctor's intense questioning included how and if I exercised. I felt certain I would "pass" this part of the questioning with an "A," because I'd been a daily walker for decades. I usually walked three miles—even at 5:00 am during my working years. He felt this was excellent, yet

---

4   "Physical activity, exercise, and physical fitness: definitions and ...." Accessed May 4, 2019. https://www.ncbi.nlm.nih.gov/pmc/articles/PMC1424733/.

I was not doing enough in other areas for good physical health. My desired "A" was really a grade of "C+" for me.

In order to live a long and healthy life, exercise on a regular basis is a must. Why? Many scientists call the lack of exercise a killing disease. Exercise delivers oxygen and nutrients to your tissues and helps your cardiovascular system work more efficiently. If you don't exercise, your muscles will become weak, your heart and lungs won't function efficiently, your joints will be susceptible to injury, and the risk of certain diseases increases, including cancer, diabetes, stroke, and heart attack.

In the US, our normal daily activities don't include much of what qualifies as physical exercise. We sit to drive, watch TV, work at a desk in an office, and so on. We would receive Olympic gold medals in sitting if those were available. We have to schedule time for exercise, which requires discipline and effort that many of us find difficult. Some people find it easier to keep moving while others struggle with it. If you have any health issues, depression, or are obese, the odds are that you're having a hard time finding the motivation to get up and move. But if you knew you could add years to your life by just getting up from your chair and walking around the house, in place or in the yard for two minutes after every 30 minutes of sitting, would you do it? Many doctors and the AHA (American Heart Association) hope you do.

Even if you are a daily exerciser, sitting for extended periods of time during your day could be a risk factor for poor health. The US Department of Health and Human

Services has released their 2nd edition of the Physical Activity Guidelines for Americans with suggested guidelines on how long to sit and when to get up and move.

These include:

- Getting up from your desk every 30 minutes
- Switching to a standing desk
- Moving around while you use your phone
- Standing up while watching TV or reading

I wish I could say my walking three miles a day covered all bases for overall fitness. However, as we age, other areas of the body need extra attention and activity to help stave off the weakening process, so the National Institutes for Health (NIH), CDC, and AHA all recommend the additional steps outlined below. We each need to take responsibility for our fitness to make sure we live our healthiest and best life.

Recommended minimum guidelines from the NIH, CDC, and AHA are broken down in three categories of aerobic exercise, strength training, and flexibility.

AEROBIC EXERCISE

Easy way to remember: 30 minutes a day, 5 times a week.

The recommendation says to engage in 150 minutes of *moderate* aerobic activity, 75 minutes of *vigorous* aerobic activity, or a combination of both per week.

As with any new activity check with your doctor before starting.

Any number of sports and cardio activities done on a regular basis will meet the minimum guidelines. Some include:

- Walking
- Tennis
- Swimming
- Biking
- Skating
- Basketball
- Running
- Hiking
- Golf (walking the course)
- Soccer
- Racquetball

Walking, my favorite activity, is one of the easiest and most effective ways to engage in the recommended aerobic activity, so it should cover everything you need if you have limited interest or ability to participate in others. For such a simple activity, it's amazing how many benefits walking offers. Regular brisk walking can help us maintain or lose weight; strengthen the immune system; prevent or manage heart disease, high blood pressure and type 2 diabetes; improve sleep; strengthen bones and muscles; improve balance and coordination; boost your mood; lower your risk of Alzheimer's and dementia; and lengthen your life.

Note on Walking: The only expense involved, which I highly recommend, is getting a good pair of walking shoes. Specialty shoe stores in most cities will take the time to measure your feet, analyze your gait, and fit you properly, so you are comfortable with a lessened chance of injury. This shouldn't mean you have to pay for the most expensive shoes in the store, if it's reputable. It's about finding the proper fit.

With my compromised immune system, I knew I had to keep to my walking routine without fail. In recent years, scientists have discovered brisk walking boosts the immune system. That led me to think I might have experienced an autoimmune outbreak much earlier in my life—or a more severe type—if I hadn't engaged in regular, sustained walking for so many years.

If you start and stay on a regular walking regimen, you will need to replace your shoes around every six months, because they will start to break down internally even though the high-tech outside doesn't show wear. Worn shoes place unequal pressure on your feet, which can impact your knees, legs, ankles, and hips. I developed groin pain on both sides and kept right on walking through the pain until I belatedly realized I should figure out what was causing it. My worn out shoes were the culprit. It took three months to right everything, so don't wear old shoes for too long like I did.

STRENGTH TRAINING

....

Easy way to remember: 2 times a week, 8-10 strength-training exercises with 8-12 repetitions of each exercise.

The US Department of Health and Human Services (DHHS) recommends strength training twice a week: 8-10 strength-training exercises, 8-12 repetitions of each exercise. Strength training strengthens muscles and helps maintain lean muscle tissue. These can be done at a gym on dedicated machines, with or without a trainer's supervision, or by using free weights and resistance bands. In addition, a host of workouts for strength training including pushups, jumping jacks, lunges, planks, and squats can be done at home or in a gym and do not require equipment. Newer studies show using lighter weights for more repetitions is as effective for building muscle as lifting heavy weights for fewer repetitions. This is good news for older adults or people new to lifting weights. Overall, pushing muscles until they're fatigued and can't lift any more offers good results.

Other activities count towards both strength training and aerobic activity and can be effective as long as you spend at least 30 minutes engaged in them.

- Heavy gardening – digging holes, planting, weeding, lifting bags of mulch, raking, etc
- Dancing
- Climbing stairs
- Shoveling

- Hill walking
- Gym classes such as boxing, rowing, Zumba, spin, and barre, pilates, TRX, and others

CHILDLIKE BEHAVIOR – JUMPING, HOPPING, SKIPPING

I was quite surprised to find out that reverting to these childhood behaviors can strengthen your bones. Osteoporosis, which is a weak bone condition, affects more than 54 million people in the US. Hip fractures, in particular, are a major health concern for older adults.

I have osteopenia, a precursor to osteoporosis, which was diagnosed with my first bone scan at 50. When I had the scan, I was told that this condition has a genetic component and that I had the additional physical type (small boned and thin) that lends itself to this. I've had two bone scans since the first. While the deterioration was minute, and no recommendation was forthcoming to start on a drug regimen, I thought I could add more to my existing routine of walking, weekly yoga, and taking calcium. Bone is a living tissue that responds to muscle work by becoming stronger. I want to avoid developing full osteoporosis, and the drugs currently prescribed for it, because the side effects alarm me.

Here are some recommendations you can do at home:

Jumping: There are techniques to use to avoid hurting yourself, such as holding onto a chair and landing with knees bent. A study done on premenopausal women doing high-impact jump training found significant

7

improvement in hip bone mineral density (BMD). The jolt of landing appears to start new bone growth, so the popular mini-trampolines will not work for this.

Hopping for two minutes a day was studied in the U.K. on a group of men over 65 which showed improvement in BMD.[5] This year-long study (called the Hip Hop study) measured the effects of hopping on one leg. The men hopped on one leg only in order to test for any differences between the two legs. Bone mapping programs showed clear BMD improvement in the leg that was used for hopping.

Skipping and balancing on one foot (as in tree pose in yoga) also puts the proper stress on your skeletal frame.

If you already incorporate tennis, hiking, cross-country skiing or snowshoeing, you may not need to add these additional activities, because these sports involve good amounts of bone-building pressure. Swimming and cycling do not increase bone density. In fact, some studies have shown they may actually *decrease* bone density levels.

I don't want to leave this section without mentioning **interval training**, which is a relatively new concept still under study for its effectiveness. Interval training applies to aerobic and strength training but is not applicable for helping with flexibility.

---

5   "Loughborough research points finds hopping can give hope to older ...." Accessed May 4, 2019. https://www.lboro.ac.uk/departments/ssehs/news/2015/loughborough-research-points-finds-hopping-can-give-hope-to-older-people.html.

INTERVAL TRAINING

Alternating burst of intense activity with intervals of lighter activity.

Newer studies show that interval training or the more intense version of High Intensity Interval Training (HIIT) may do an enormous amount—down to our very cells—to erase what the years have done to our bodies. This technique can be incorporated into any of your exercise routines. If walking, for instance, alternate very fast walking with regular-paced walking. Or in a cycle (spin) class, alternate intense pace cycling with slower speeds.

Cell Metabolism published a study conducted by the Mayo Clinic in 2017[6] that showed both younger and older test subjects participating in interval training experienced the strongest increases in gene activity compared to other types of exercise. Gene activity included increased mitochondrial function (known as the powerhouses of the cell), increased skeletal muscle function, and enhancement of ribosomal proteins. This gene activity reversed some signs of aging. The study was conducted on 72 healthy, sedentary men and women who were either 30 or younger or older than 64 utilizing HIIT, resistance training (RT), and combined exercise training for 12 weeks.

In fact, the older group experienced an even higher increase in cell activity than the younger group, suggesting

---

6   "Enhanced Protein Translation Underlies Improved ...-Cell Press." 7 Mar. 2017, https://www.cell.com/cell-metabolism/pdfExtended/S1550-4131(17)30099-2. Accessed 12 Jun. 2019.

that older people's cells responded to interval training in such a way as to erase years of damage to older muscles.

Due to this and other studies on the benefits of HIIT, I'm considering adding the fast/slow walking to complement my routine.

Scientists don't fully understand yet how these positive results happened—as is similar with other medical advances, it takes time to find the why—but I'm learning to read, decipher, and decide whether to act on the new information without the full explanations at hand. In general, these are low risk ways to possibly improve your health.

FLEXIBILITY

Easy way to remember: Two times per week.

Flexibility exercises are recommended twice a week and can include yoga, stretching, and/or Tai Chi. Benefits of flexibility exercises improve functional abilities and athletic performance. A stretched and lengthened muscle achieves full range of motion more easily. Daily tasks such as reaching, bending, or stooping are improved and leave less possibility for injury. When muscles are more flexible, the body's circulation improves its ability to carry nutrients and oxygen throughout.

TAI CHI

Tai Chi (also known as "tai chi chuan") originated in China many centuries ago and has become increasingly popular in the US. Most of the versions practiced in the US today are a modified version of the original. This ancient form of Chinese martial art, today practiced as a slow-moving meditative exercise, helps reduce stress and increase flexibility, balance, muscle strength, energy and stamina, among others. Although it helps aerobically, it doesn't help enough to rely solely on this activity for aerobic exercise. In the *Journal of Sport and Health Science*, recent studies were analyzed and reported findings that Tai Chi has a positive impact on memory and learning, and lessens anxiety symptoms.

You can often find classes offered in communities, including many senior centers in larger metropolitan areas. It should be taught by someone with proper training, look for certification through the ATCQA (American Tai Chi and Qigong Association). Check out your local community colleges, community centers, and YMCAs for availability. Tai Chi is low impact and generally safe for all ages.

Tai Chi is especially good for strengthening the body to reduce the chance of falling. How many of us know of older people who fall and break a hip, which leads to complications and even death? Tai Chi helps improve balance by targeting all the physical components needed to stay upright—leg strength, flexibility, range of motion, and reflexes—which tend to decline with age.

Tai Chi also makes you more aware of both your internal body and the external world. This gives you a better sense of your position in space, so you won't be as likely to trip and fall when, for instance, you're walking while talking on your phone. This sense of your position in space is called "proprioception," which OxfordDictionaries.com defines as *the perception or awareness of the position and movement of the body.* Far more activities rely on a good sense of proprioception than we think about on a daily basis. When we sit, stand, or bend, we're using our proprioceptive system. The same holds true when climbing stairs, using escalators, lifting and carrying boxes, and walking in darkness. Hobbies such as painting, dancing, and sports such as tennis and golf, also use proprioception. It's important in our everyday lives.

Along with increased proprioception, Tai Chi has an additional integral piece that involves interaction with your inner spirit. It is called "Qi," which is the vital life force and energy that flows through the body's energy pathways. Qi is accessed by the slow deliberate movements, meditation, and breathing exercises of Tai Chi. In TCM (Traditional Chinese Medicine), the goal is to have Qi flowing smoothly throughout the body. Good health will be present when those conditions exist. When it doesn't, TCM practitioners recommend changes in diet, herbal remedies, acupuncture, and Tai Chi.

Although I have taken many Tai Chi classes, I admit I'm not currently enrolled as I write this. Some habits stick and some do not. It is not available in my mountain community where I am in the summer, which certainly gives me somewhat of an excuse while I'm there. However, it's readily available in Florida where I spend winters. I am reminded I should be more disciplined and return to it.

YOGA

> *Yoga is a Hindu spiritual and ascetic discipline, a part of which, including breath control, simple meditation and the adoption of specific bodily postures, is widely practised for health and relaxation. (Oxforddictionaries.com)*

Yoga originated in India at least 5,000 years ago and has achieved a growing popularity in the US where you can find a style to suit most any preference and health status. Recent studies indicate regular yoga practice can provide a wide range of benefits both mental and physical, including:

- Sleep problems
- Losing weight
- Flexibility
- Bone strength
- Reducing arthritis pain
- Strengthening your immune system
- Improving cardio and circulatory health
- Symptoms of menopause
- Managing and improving symptoms from some chronic diseases such as COPD, MS, diabetes, IBS
- Depression and anxiety

- Improving general health and energy
- Back pain
- Improving symptoms of some cancers

I enjoy my yoga classes. While I'm not proficient in the practice, it still seems to have a calming effect and is tremendous for stretching. The benefits related to flexibility, bone strength, and strengthening my immune system keep me coming back. I've been able to incorporate it into my weekly schedule while in Florida but haven't found the right type of class where I am in the summer. If you're like me at all, self- discipline is tough, and I need the structure of a class and teacher to continue while others utilize the many online options available.

According to the 2017 National Health Interview Survey (NHIS), the use of yoga in the US has increased a significant amount in the last few years from 9.5% in 2012 to 14.3% in 2017.[7] More people are incorporating yoga in their overall health plans due to its perceived many benefits.

Some of the most popular yoga types in the US are Hatha Yoga, Iyengar Yoga, Ashtanga Yoga, Vinyasa Yoga, Bikram or hot yoga, and Kundalini Yoga. For those with health issues that don't allow for standing unaided for any length of time or full body stretching, a modified version called chair yoga can be beneficial. This is offered in many regular yoga class centers, in senior fitness centers, retirement facilities, and others.

7   "National Health Interview Survey 2017 | NCCIH." 14 Nov. 2018, https://nccih.nih.gov/research/statistics/NHIS/2017. Accessed 11 May. 2019.

Yoga has been part of my regular schedule for four years. At the insistence of friends, I tried it a dozen years ago, but it wasn't for me at that time. I was either trying the wrong type of class or had an instructor who didn't fit well with me. An alternative healing practitioner suggested I return to yoga. I attend a weekly yoga class, which is gentle and incorporates elements of hatha yoga. It's run by an excellent instructor named Ellen Riordan, PhD, LMT, who has become a friend of mine.

For those who are worried about the religious connotation of yoga and whether practicing yoga means going against their particular belief system, there are ways to adjust your practice. While yoga's roots are in an eastern religion, the repackaging in the US has meant the practice is heavily into the physical movements along with breathing techniques rather than as a spiritual practice.

We must stay active to keep our bodies operating the way they should, and it is difficult to fulfill the recommended guidelines with any single activity. Our ancestors were hunter gatherers. Our bodies function much the same as in the Stone Age with our systems operating most efficiently when physically active. The modern world and its advances make it easy for us to move as little as possible and that causes enormous risk to our health. For our systems to perform well, we must take charge and incorporate at least moderate exercise.

EAT A HEALTHY
BALANCED DIET

D IET. WHAT AN INFLAMMATORY WORD. People's eyes either glaze over at the mention of it or light up with anticipation that this could be the answer to their health and weight issues. The problem with it is built right into the dictionary definition at Oxforddictionaries.com.

1. The kinds of food that a person, animal, or community habitually eats.

or

2. A special course of food to which a person restricts themselves, either to lose weight or for medical reasons.

This is all about definition number one and *not* about definition number two. Even the mention of the word "diet" in the context of restrictive behavior or forbidden foods makes me crave those foods. In general, nutrition experts believe diets that restrict people—unless medically advised—are only temporary solutions and will not solve long-term health issues.

In my research on diets to live healthier and longer, every single reputable source (Harvard, NIH, Mayo Clinic, AHA, USDA, DHHS, FDA, and *New England Journal of Medicine*) mentioned the Mediterranean Diet. Even so, no long-term, unbiased study clearly shows that one diet or another ranks as the best. Many studies over decades show the Mediterranean Diet has consistent health benefits. I'll review its overall guidelines here.

THE MEDITERRANEAN DIET AND WHY FOOD MATTERS

A healthy, strong body fights off disease better than an unhealthy one. This means that the food we put into our bodies is crucial to how well our body systems work, and sticking to a Mediterranean diet might slow down aging. A 2016 EU-funded project tested 1,142 participants, all over the age of 65, from five different European countries (France, Italy, Poland, the Netherlands, and the UK), on a Mediterranean diet. The participants showed a significant reduction in the C-reactive protein, which is one of the main inflammatory markers linked with the aging process.

Additional studies show that the Mediterranean diet might reduce risks related to heart attack and breast cancer while possibly lowering the risk of dementia. Brain health, in general, might be significantly improved according to a study analyzing the diets of 400 adults (73-76 years old in Scotland over a three-year period).[8] MRI scans were done to analyze overall brain volume and thickness of the brain's cortex. The researchers found that those who closely followed a Mediterranean diet were less likely to lose brain volume as they aged when compared with those who didn't follow such a diet. More research is needed to determine the effect this diet might have on degenerative brain disease risk, but this still suggests that we are all better off by following some version of it.

The Mediterranean Diet emphasizes fruits, vegetables, fish, whole grains, and healthy fats with many differences between the countries of origin. The Greeks, Italians, Spanish and French all have their own version with a common denominator being to eat as organically as possible.

- Eat 5 – 10 servings a day of fruits and vegetables.
- Eat healthy fats, including olive oil, avocado, or coconut oil, and avoid butter unless it is organic, preferably from grass-fed sources. The diet does not include butter substitutes.
- Whole grains – bread, cereal, rice and pasta products with "whole" as the major emphasis. Whole grains have all three original parts: the bran, germ, and endosperm that they had when the grain was growing in the fields. Refined grains have had some of those removed.

---

8   "Mediterranean-type diet and brain structural change from 73 to ...-NCBI." Accessed May 5, 2019. https://www.ncbi.nlm.nih.gov/pmc/articles/PMC5278943/.

- Seeds, nuts, and legumes at least twice a week.
- Eggs (organic if possible), cheese (not processed and aged is preferred), and yogurt (without added sugar or artificial flavors).
- Fish, poultry, and lean pork twice a week. Top fish choices being salmon (wild if possible), mackerel, sardines, albacore tuna, although many other fish have benefits as well.
- Red meat should be limited to no more than a few times a month.
- Desserts that are sugar based no more than a few times a month.
- Drink red wine in moderation (US recommendation one glass a day for women, two for men).
- Limit refined starches, added sugars, processed and fried foods, and avoid excessive salt intake.

Sounds simple right? Maybe for some. I continue to struggle with a portion of this. I don't eat enough in one category while eating too much in another, and I can't seem to eliminate potato chips and mayonnaise from my diet.

My alternative doctor, Dr. Patton, questioned me about my eating habits in great detail during my initial consultation. At the time, it seemed unusual and certainly not part of what you would expect from a Western traditional doctor. I didn't realize it then, but this is common with alternative or TCM (Traditional Chinese Medicine) doctors. In general, Western medicine treats symptoms and individual organs while Eastern tries to find the root cause before treatment and treats the whole body.

While I thought I had a fairly balanced diet, he saw room for improvement and recommended I eat as much organic food as possible, add as many greens as I could handle in each day, add more fruit, and cut down on red meat. While I didn't eat that much processed food, he still wanted me to eliminate chips or at least cut them down to a minimum. If I had a glass of wine, I was supposed to have it with a meal.

The CDC recommends no more than one glass of wine a day for women and two for men. This is the most restrictive recommendation among developed countries. A US study released in 2018 contends that no amount is safe (this was a meta-analysis of data from nearly 700 studies worldwide from University of Washington Institute for Health Metrics and Evaluation 2016 Global Burden of Disease Study). However, as of this writing, experts are calling the extremely broad scope of the analysis into question, because it did not allow for specificity of countries, populations, or differentiation of types of alcohol nor did it address any proven health benefits. The decision is yours on which guidelines to follow.

ORGANIC

In the discussion around healthy eating, this topic comes up a lot. As I indicated earlier, Dr. Patton recommended I incorporate as much organic food as possible into my diet. In the process, I thought I knew all about organics, yet some research showed me I had a bit to learn, including just what that all-important USDA organic label means.

21

What does organic mean exactly?

Food produced without synthetic fertilizers or pesticides and free from chemical injections or additives, such as antibiotics or hormones, can be considered organic. Organic produce has more nutrition than conventionally raised foods and no concern over side effects from chemicals. Organics have a reputation for being expensive and, personally, I have found that to be mostly true. However, with the larger grocery chains adding their own organic brand, I've noticed decreased prices. The cheapest way to obtain organics is to grow them yourself using natural fertilizers and no chemical pesticides, but not everyone wants to do that or can.

Farmers markets are a good place for fresh quality produce but they may or may not be certified organic. A small farm may not have the resources to obtain the certification. Your personal knowledge of the individual farm and what they are utilizing on their crops should be the deciding factor in what you purchase. I was driving 25 minutes to a local co-op that provided access for certified organic farms until a certified organic farmer set up a booth in the farmers market five minutes away from me. Before that, I had no reliable knowledge of treatment of crops from the other farms represented at farmers markets.

Certified organic. The most important word in that statement is *certified*. Anything that has passed the USDA (United States Department of Agriculture) organic standards has a green and white seal somewhere on the labeling that says "USDA organic." If there is no green seal, the food has not passed the USDA organic standards. The USDA.gov site states:

Organic certification requires that farmers and handlers document their processes and undergo inspections every year. Organic on-site inspections account for every component of the operation, including, but not limited to seed sources: soil conditions, crop health, weed and pest management, water systems, inputs, contamination and co-mingling risks and prevention, and record-keeping. Tracing organic products from start to finish is part of the USDA organic promise.[9]

That is the admirable mission statement of the USDA. The reality is there are reported problems with the organic certification, everything from third-party inspectors hired by the farmers, which is allowed, but raises concerns over impartiality to inspections happening infrequently with simply not enough manpower to vet all the businesses. The situation isn't perfect, yet it's the only system we have in place to monitor organics.

In addition, misleading food labeling leads consumers to believe they are buying certified organic products when they're not. Even though stricter labeling regulations have passed into law, more are needed. "Natural," "cage free," "free range," and many others are marketing phrases and do not mean the product is organic. Look for the USDA label. To further confuse the consumer, the beef industry

9   "Organic 101: What the USDA Organic Label Means |
USDA." Accessed May 5, 2019. https://www.usda.gov/media/
blog/2012/03/22/organic-101-what-usda-organic-label-means.

now produces and labels beef with designations such as organic, grass fed, and grass finished.

Experts agree that **organic 100% grass fed** with no grain of any kind is the healthiest beef to eat with the highest nutritional content. Unfortunately, it is the hardest to find and the most expensive at this point.

- An **organic** label means the cows were fed grain, which is certified organic when not feeding on grass or hay, and farms must certify no pesticides or chemical fertilizers were used on the land for the prior three years. Further, no antibiotics or growth-enhancing hormones may be used. The designation does not differentiate how much grain versus grass is fed to cows.
- A **grass fed** label means the cattle were fed on grass or hay at some point in their grazing life. Additions of grain, with the standard being corn, are possible at any point with this label. And the grass, hay, or grain could have had pesticides applied or antibiotics or hormones administered to the cattle unless it states otherwise. Currently, no USDA labeling standard exists for grass fed, meaning the cattle could have been grass fed for a week and then moved right back to eating corn grain. 100% grass fed is the key to guarantee no grain was added.
- **Grass finished versus grain finished**. Traditional beef production sends cattle to market where there is a period of months where they are "finished" before being sold. Typically, this means they are in a feed lot and fed corn grain to rapidly add weight. If

the beef is labeled grass finished, it means the cattle remained on grass until being sold.

Why the high cost for grass fed or organic versus traditional feed lot cattle? It's much more expensive for the ranchers, especially where grass finishing is concerned. It's a longer process to fatten cattle to acceptable market weight on wild grasses. And if organic is involved, there are extra expenses in adhering to proper procedures. For many, it is economics driving the feeding of cattle for the rancher. You generally will see limited availability of the premium product, namely organic and or 100% grass fed.

The takeaway is read your labels or find out the procedures of the farms if you are buying at local farmers markets.

WATER

Most of us do not drink enough water. To function properly, all cells and organs need water. In fact, the Earth's surface is 71% water, and 70% of the human body is comprised of water. While certain foods have a higher water content, such as tomatoes or soups, we need to drink water in order to get enough. A general consensus among medical experts indicates we need to drink half of our body weight in ounces every day. An example would be your weight (150lbs) x .05 = 75 oz. of water per day.

You can get fluid into your system through non-water sources, such as juices or milk, but milk is not an option for many adults, and juices can have added sugar or other ingredients. Coffee, tea, and alcohol act as diuretics to some degree, which is the opposite of what our bodies need. Recent studies indicate sodas, especially diet soda, contain a host of other ingredients, including artificial sweeteners, phosphoric acid, potassium benzoate, artificial coloring, and caffeine. Many medical sources suggest caution and limited use. In addition, "exercise" drinks can contain additional sugars or sugar substitutes. Read labels to see what you're really drinking.

Proper water consumption helps with digestion, sharpness of mind, skin, appetite, and joint and muscle pain. The negative consequences of not drinking enough water can directly affect the kidneys. Kidneys remove waste products from the body and, without enough liquid, you may be putting yourself at risk of kidney disease or kidney failure. Other possible negative effects are circulatory problems, increased blood sugar, and digestion problems.

How to ensure you are getting enough healthy plain water?

Sadly, it's not as simple as turning on your tap. In some areas, tap water contains unsafe amounts of arsenic, aluminum, and even traces of prescription and OTC drugs. To do some research, visit the EPA website and check out your particular area, because they are responsible for overseeing the quality of your tap water. The federal government requires tap water to be tested regularly and, in big cities, disinfected, filtered, and tested for various bacteria. The results are public, and you should be able to access them through your local government site if you are not sent an annual water report. Depending on the area, these reports can be difficult to read. A local government contact in your area may be able to give you any information you need on your local water quality.

If an individual's source of water is a well, not a public water system, the well should be regularly tested by the owner because no overseeing government body checks individual wells.

The consistent advice from experts is to filter your water. Options include everything from a full in-home system, such as an RO (reverse osmosis) system to simple carbon filters by Brita and PUR. The need for filtration applies whether you have city tap water or well water. We are on well water in Colorado, and it's been tested a number of times. Since the water quality isn't good, we took our builder's recommendation and installed a RO system.

Bottled water would seem to be a safer choice, but a fairly high percentage of bottled water actually consists of tap water (sometimes filtered and sometimes not) from unknown sources. The FDA is responsible for ensuring the safety and truthful labeling of bottled water sold nationally. If it is sold and packaged within a state, the state is responsible for regulating water. There have been studies done (NIH) which are critical of the FDA regulations on bottled water, feeling they are too lenient and given low priority for safety inspections. In short, check your primary source of drinking water, filter your water, limit diuretic sources, and drink the recommended amount of every day.

SUPPLEMENTS

Ideally, *eat your vitamins*. Experts agree that supplements cannot replace the nutrition in food. Don't make the mistake of thinking you can get your full dose of nutrition by taking a handful of supplements and then eating whatever and whenever you want. We take a multitude of supplements without realizing it's a huge industry ($37 billion) with few government regulations. I've greatly reduced the number of supplements I take. After researching them further, I discovered many of them were likely ineffective while costing a great deal.

The FDA defines supplements as products "intended to add further nutritional value to (supplement) the diet." They aren't defined as drugs, so they don't fall under normal FDA guidelines. They can intervene only if a supplement has been shown to cause significant harm to a person's health, "adverse events" as the FDA calls them, or is found to include banned substances or unapproved new drugs. A 2016 study published in the *New England Journal of Medicine* estimated that 23,000 emergency room visits a year were linked to supplements. Use caution in both choosing and using supplements.

When you seek out supplements, you may be surprised by the size of the supplement section in most stores that carry them. The industry has almost 6,000 companies producing close to 75,000 products. The consumer's problem is determining what's in these products and if they are beneficial or harmful to your health.

This section is not meant as a guide to what supplements to purchase. The large number of products would require an entire book on its own. I would suggest looking at Webmd.com, Mayo Clinic or other reputable sites online for specifics on individual supplements.

Factors to look out for when buying a supplement.

- If it is not a certified organic product, don't buy if it doesn't have a complete list of ingredients. There could be other unknown substances included.
- Be cautious if the supplement was made outside the US. Standards may not be the same.
- Check if the product is on the recall list. The recall list is on the FDA website under "food."
- Check to make sure there is no interaction between the supplement and any medication you're taking.
- Take only the dose recommended and watch for any side effects.
- Check whether the supplement has bioavailability, meaning the body's ability to absorb the nutrient. Many of these nutrients have limited bioavailability in supplement form and, most likely, that information will not be on the bottle labeling. Search on reputable sites such as WebMD, NIH, or MayoClinic for supplement information
- Check with your doctor before adding any supplements.

Multivitamins

Even the ubiquitous multivitamins are suspect these days. Long-term studies using a multivitamin versus a placebo showed no difference in heart disease, delayed death from any cause, or brain cognitive functions in the various test participants. Many physicians versed in nutrition believe most people get the recommended daily vitamins from their normal diet. Unless you have a condition that warrants vitamin supplements, you may have no need to take one. I have taken a multivitamin for years and am strongly considering whether to continue. Check with your physician before making a change.

After reviewing a number of large long term studies on the efficacy of multivitamins, scientists for the US Preventive Services Task Force concluded no clear evidence existed that multivitamins added any benefits. The issue with multivitamins is complicated by the fact that there is no standard, and multivitamins have a varying nutrient list along with individual differing strengths. While some primary care doctors still recommend taking a regular strength multivitamin daily as an insurance policy despite the well publicized studies, they are *not* recommending taking multivitamins labeled "mega" or "extra strength," which exceeds the Recommended Daily Allowance (RDA). The RDA is produced and updated periodically by the Food And Nutrition Board of the National Research Council/ National Academy of Sciences. Combined with vitamins naturally occurring in your food, taking too much could be a prescription for trouble.

Probiotics

For the past three years, I've taken a probiotic. I suspect you've heard the word and seen it slapped on labels for every type of product whether it's edible or not. Probiotics are commonly known as "good bacteria." They are live cultures that help kill off bad bacteria in your gut, reducing infection. Some doctors now recommend patients take probiotics along with a course of antibiotics, because antibiotics kill off both good and bad bacteria, which could cause additional infections.

Various studies indicate gut health is crucial to good health overall. Previously, I thought probiotics were all about helping a sluggish digestion. While that is part of it, studies indicate we're only at the beginning of the discovery process about probiotic benefits. A growing body of scientific evidence suggests probiotics help with allergy symptoms, vaginal and urinary tract infections, IBS, skin and hair quality, H. pylori (the cause of ulcers), cold and flu, anxiety, weight loss, recurrence of bladder cancer, and immune function. They may even act as a counter to the toxicity we are bombarded with on a daily basis. Some doctors think probiotics could become a daily recommended requirement in the near future.

We do not know exactly how much and what types do the most good. I take a tablet that contains 10 types of live bacteria in a 30 billion quantity, and I chose it after researching what was out there. It sounds like a lot, but consider that we have trillions of bacteria living in our gut.

Why am I taking a tablet rather than getting the pro-biotics in food? The foods that contain a significant amount of probiotics would require that I eat/drink a huge amount of those foods every day and I know myself well enough to know that's not going to happen. A daily tablet is something I can consistently take.

What to keep in mind if you plan to add probiotic foods.

Live cultures are all important. Read the labels to confirm the cultures are live and to determine the amount and types of bacteria, and buy organic when you can. In the case of yogurt, as an example, much has been processed beyond recognition. You're better off buying plain live culture yogurt and adding your own fruits. In the case of kombucha (fermented tea), there is enormous controversy over the different kinds of products available. Kombucha comes as either heat pasteurized (thereby killing the live cultures) or raw (using something called the symbiotic culture of bacteria and yeast), which does not use heat to stop the fermentation process. Ongoing legal battles between the two factions may one day cause the industry to use a new standard in labeling. In the meantime, if you are buying kombucha for the purpose of adding probiotics, look for the words "live cultures."

Keep in mind that the myriad of products using the word "probiotic" in their marketing and packaging may not have live cultures, and no standard has been set regarding quantity. This means there could be a very small amount added, which is not enough to make a difference in your health.

> **Probiotics occur naturally in:** Kimchi, cottage cheese, kombucha (raw unpasteurized), live cultured yogurt, sauerkraut (unpasteurized), miso, pickles (in salt and water, no vinegar), kefir, apple cider vinegar (raw and unpasteurized), and tempeh.

Overall, try to eat a diet of mostly minimally processed foods with a strong emphasis on vegetables, fruits, and whole grains and stay away from too much protein, salt, sugar, and the "bad" fats. Make sure to drink your recommended amount of water daily, choose supplements wisely, and read the labels, and check with your doctor before making any changes. You'll be way ahead on the road to good health.

MANAGE STRESS

Stress is defined as: a state of mental or emotional strain or tension resulting from adverse or very demanding circumstances. Oxford dictionaries.com

WITH MY FIRST HAIR LOSS event, I did not correlate stress as a factor in the equation at all. In fact, I went an entire year without making *any* changes in my lifestyle. Remember, I thought that the culprit was the temporary use of an estrogen cream. Only after my second hair loss event, after having been hit over the head so to speak, did I realize something else was happening.

As I took tests to measure stress, Dr. Patton warned me the results were probably going to show elevated levels of cortisol (the fight or flight hormone), and he would prescribe treatment from there. When my results came back from the lab, they were so extreme that the lab called Dr. Patton to inquire if the patient (me) had followed the instructions correctly. They wanted to do a retest at no charge as soon as possible. I rushed my saliva samples to the office as if they were an organ ready for transport to save a life. Maybe I was in denial over the seriousness of my condition, but everyone's reaction seemed pretty alarmist.

The retest returned with the same perturbing results. As Dr. Patton told me later he had rarely, in his many years of practice, seen anything that severe. When he had, the patient had additional serious health conditions requiring a referral to a specialist. And here I was, seemingly healthy as a horse, yet heading towards becoming a bald one.

He started me on a whole treatment plan which involved:

- Weekly acupuncture (new for me)
- A regimen of cortisol-reducing natural supplements
- Advice to start meditation (also my first experience)
- Increased organics and greens in my food
- Reduced intake of processed foods
- Limiting alcohol to a glass of wine with dinner
- Avoiding violent media (books, movies, TV)

He wanted me to spend some time thinking about my past, my relationships and my belief systems, so a weekly counseling session was included as well. This felt overwhelming and was the opposite of the Western medicine approach I'd experienced before. I came from a family who were "sweep-it-under-the-rug" and "fix-yourself-and-never-ask-for-help" kind of people. For decades, I followed that path as a highly functioning independent adult, so I was surprised to find I had carried unproductive thought processes and that they helped perpetuate stress reactions. Your thoughts can manifest into physical symptoms.

Chronic stress has been shown to have negative health impacts and age exacerbates it. Diseases and disorders linked to chronic stress include autoimmune, depression, anxiety, heart issues, diabetes, and some forms of cancer. It can even affect our bone density. NIH states: "Chronic psychological stress is a risk factor for osteoporosis." [10]

Since we are all individuals with different adaptive traits, know that some techniques may work better than others for reducing stress. Try some out and see what, if any, have a positive impact for you.

SLEEP

Dr. Patton questioned me on my sleep patterns. That was one area that did not seem to top the list on my issues. Most nights my sleep was 8 ½ to 9 hours—not completely undisturbed but with only a brief waking. I knew many people who were not able to have a significant amount of undisturbed sleep and suffered.

---

10   "Chronic Psychological Stress as a Risk Factor of Osteoporosis.-NCBI." Accessed May 5, 2019. https://www.ncbi.nlm.nih.gov/pubmed/26667192.

Poor sleep has been linked to medical problems such as obesity, diabetes, cancer, immune deficiency, high blood pressure, memory and cognitive performance, and even increased skin aging. Getting enough sleep is considered to be important for total body restitution like energy conservation, thermoregulation (maintenance of constant internal temperature), and tissue recovery.

Exciting recent discoveries by an NIH funded study show an even more imperative reason for good quality sleep. The study suggests the brain has a "housekeeping" function that flushes out toxins during sleep that build up during waking hours.[11] This could have significant implications for various neurological disorders such as Alzheimer's and cardiovascular issues. More studies are underway as of this writing.

What does good sleep mean to you?

There is no absolute right amount of sleep, but current recommendations from the National Sleep Foundation are in agreement that adults need a minimum of seven hours every night.

What may help for unbroken sleep:

- Stick to a regular bedtime – go to sleep and get up at the same time each day, even on weekends.

---

11   "Sleep Drives Metabolite Clearance from the Adult Brain–NCBI–NIH." 18 Oct. 2013, https://www.ncbi.nlm.nih.gov/pmc/articles/PMC3880190/. Accessed 9 May. 2019.

- Take time to unwind – turn off TV and other electronic devices an hour before bed and listen to music or read a book.
- Don't drink alcohol close to bedtime as it may make it harder to stay asleep.
- Don't ingest caffeine late in the day – it's found in coffee, tea, sodas, and chocolate.
- Avoid napping late in the afternoon or evening.
- Have a regular exercise routine but don't exercise within 3 hrs of your bedtime.
- Stay active during the day. Keep your body and mind moving.
- As a temporary measure, using over-the-counter sleep aids or prescription medicines may help you sleep. These should be used for a short duration only, are not a cure for insomnia and may be habit forming.

MEDITATION

Meditate–to focus one's mind for a period of time, in silence or with the aid of chanting, for religious or spiritual purposes or as a method of relaxation. (Oxforddictionaries.com)

When I started meditation practice, Dr. Patton told me to sit on the floor or in a chair, and not lie down as I would just go to sleep. I was to set a timer for 10 minutes at first. He told me to make up a mantra—a few words or sounds but not recognizable words—to use as a silent chant to try and quiet my mind and stop all those pesky thoughts from creeping in. I was skeptical and told him so. I was quite sure I wouldn't be any good at this meditation thing. After all, I was type A and impatient. He said it didn't matter and that even if I meditated "badly," I'd have started something that would bring positive change. This goes far deeper than your normal senses of sight, hearing, smell, touch, and taste. It requires digging down below the surface and sitting with yourself. You become still, aware of your core self, peaceful and centered, and your connection with the universe.

During the first few months, I counted quiet in seconds—not minutes. Every noise was a distraction. But I persisted, and things changed. I was able to have increasingly more time in absolute silence in my mind. That is the place you aim for according to experts in the field (Jon Kabat-Zinn, Eckhart Tolle, Jack Kornfield, Dr. Rick Hanson, Daniel Siegel, Deepak Chopra, Sara Lazar, and many others). I realize there are many people out there who wish to start a meditation practice and just can't seem to be motivated to begin. I was definitely in that same group and might not have ever started but for the doctor telling me to do it for my health. I'm amazed that I'm now a daily meditator, and I do not plan on ever stopping. These days, I can meditate in a variety of environments, which are noisy and filled with people, including on planes. This feels like a major accomplishment. I try and stay present as much as I can every day and believe I handle the stresses of life much better than before. People close to me say I seem calmer, and it really feels that way. I still have my moments, but I'm able to let emotions filter through me most of the time. I stop and realize the emotion is there and do not let it define how I take action. Situations that would have sent my blood pressure rising to the ceiling and caused me to see red now seem relatively harmless and I watch in a detached way—as if outside of myself.

If you have not explored meditation up to this point and are rolling your eyes over just the mention of the word, understand there are proven health benefits from this that may help you live longer and better. Traditional medicine has now embraced meditation, and all the scientific studies confirm it has enormous benefits to our bodies and minds. Study after study indicates that meditation is beneficial to our health. It has even been introduced to at-risk school curriculums with positive results, including reduced violent behavior, less illness and absenteeism, and higher test scores. Our modern technology now gives scientists the ability to see actual changes in the brain of practiced meditators versus those who don't. Magnetic resonance imaging (MRI) is used to measure cortical thickness of the brain. Thinning of the cortical thickness is a negative consequence of aging, depression, and other conditions. In simple terms thicker is better. A number of studies have confirmed neural degeneration is substantially less in regular meditators.[12] We may even be able to alter our individual brain structure through meditation. Studies measuring cortical thickness of the brain's gray and white matter in practiced meditators and non-meditators of different ages found the meditators'

---

12 "Mindfulness practice leads to increases in regional brain gray matter ...." Accessed May 5, 2019. https://www.ncbi.nlm.nih.gov/pmc/articles/PMC3004979/.

thickness much greater. In my words, a much younger appearing brain.

Meditation has emerged from a "new age" practice to rapidly become part of mainstream society. While the emphasis is new, it is an ancient practice with archaeologists and scholars in agreement that it is probably over 5,000 years old. Meditation appears in texts in all the world's major religions: Judaism, Buddhism, Hindu, Christian, Muslim, and others. Meditation does not have to be associated with religion, however. It is a mind and body practice that you can use for whatever purpose suits you the best.

According to the National Institutes of Health, most meditative practices have four elements in common:

- A quiet location with as few distractions as possible
- A specific, comfortable posture (sitting, lying down, walking, or in other positions)
- A focus of attention (a specially chosen word or set of words, an object, or the sensations of the breath)
- An open attitude (letting distractions come and go naturally without judging them)

There are clear signs that indicate meditation is beneficial to the human body and mind. There have been literally thousands of scientific studies done on meditation in the last 60 years, with the most compelling studies done during the last decade due to the invention of the modern instruments (fMRI and EEG). These instruments allow scientists to study brain changes before and after meditation making for clearer analysis on the effects of meditation. Even so, science does not have a full understanding of *why* meditation seems to work. I say *why* doesn't matter. Just do it.

Some of the benefits of meditation:

1. Reduction of stress
2. Possible slowing of cellular aging
3. Better sleep
4. Reduction of depression and anxiety
5. Reduce blood pressure
6. Boosted immune system
7. Reduced pain
8. Improved IBS and ulcerative colitis

Hundreds of CEOs, celebrities, sports figures, and other high profile people have meditated for years while keeping the fact quiet until it became more socially acceptable. The list includes: Derek Jeter, George Lucas, Rupert Murdoch, Paul McCartney, Arianna Huffington, Kobe Bryant, Tom Hanks, Edward Saatchi, Martin Scorsese, Oprah Winfrey, Russell Simmons, George Stephanopoulos, Lebron James, Howard Stern, Barry Zito, Michael Jordan, and Nicole Kidman to name just a few.

Studies show meditation might slow cellular aging. Meditation seems to lengthen the telomeres in our bodies. Telomeres are "protective protein caps" at the end of our DNA strands that allow for continued cell replication. Longer telomeres mean the cells replicate more and, therefore, lengthen lifespan. A shorter telomere length in cells is linked with poorer immune system functioning, degenerative conditions (such as osteoporosis and Alzheimer's disease), and cardiovascular disease.[13] This happens naturally as we age yet can be accelerated by stress.

All of this exciting information indicates that we might be able to make a difference in how we age—mentally and physically—by doing a short daily meditation. My daily morning walk has morphed into an additional type of meditation. It sets up my day to be open and positive, and I feel better the more I do it.

As to types of meditation, there are an endless range of practices. What all of them have in common is a way to shift your consciousness inward and become still, shutting out the external world. I have committed to a 20-minute daily practice that I rarely stray from. I enthusiastically endorse it to anyone who will listen, because it's been a positive influence on my life. To choose a practice, realize there's no one correct way. My advice would be to start with something simple and short in duration, and don't pay a substantial amount of money. There is simply too much out there that works and is free or minimal cost.

You may have heard of TM (Transcendental Meditation). It is a type of meditation that was made famous in the 60s when the Beatles discovered it in India with its founder Maharishi. It is the only meditation technique I'm aware

---

13   "Maintaining the End: Roles of Telomere Proteins in End ...–NCBI–NIH." Accessed May 5, 2019. https://www.ncbi.nlm.nih.gov/pmc/articles/PMC3256267/.

44

of that charges a substantial fee that you can't learn on your own. There is a "secret" element involved so it is difficult to delve deep enough into what's it all about, and there are endless naysayers who have left this practice behind. I don't see any reason to try TM myself as I've gotten so much out of my own meditation technique. Meditation in whatever form seems to have great mental and physical health benefits. Your individual commitment to a meditation practice seems to be the key here. Just do it.

MY SIMPLE MEDITATION PRACTICE

I go to a quiet place and sit on the floor with a cushion or on carpet in a traditional yogic crossed legs position. I sit where I can brace my back if I get tired.

1. I set a timer for 20 minutes.
2. I close my eyes and do what's called a body scan, which is simply focusing on each part of my body and then releasing before I let the quiet come into my mind.

That simple daily practice has improved how I process stress. I believe it's one of the most important things I do each day.

Meditation has taken me into another realm that I'm still trying to understand. Every once in a while, along with the struggle to quiet my mind, meditation will become a strange place where words are spoken to me or a vision of me being in another time and place appears. Over the last four years, I've stopped using the mantra word and allowed my mind to come on its own to a quiet place. In that space I've had some pretty astounding experiences, such as messages coming from some ethereal space to what felt like visions of some sort. Those experiences are rare in my world, most days the practice serves to simply calm and center me.

BREATHING

Obviously, we can't live without this. Breathing falls under the category of automatic systems in our bodies that we don't have to think about much. Specific types of breathing have different names: belly breathing, paced respiration, abdominal breathing, and diaphragmatic breathing. They all have deep breathing in common and bring extra oxygen into your body.

Many of us are not doing deep breathing. Instead, we engage in shallow chest breathing without even being aware of it and that can lead to cardiovascular episodes, premature aging, tiredness, tight muscles, digestive disturbances, and autoimmune conditions. A reaction to any kind of stress, can trigger the sympathetic nervous system (the "fight or flight" response), which can cause faster shortened breath. If this happens continually throughout a person's day, it becomes a bad habit that we may barely notice.

Deep breathing involves breathing in slowly through your nose and filling your lungs and lower stomach. Your belly will expand and rise. This type of breathing can slow the heartbeat, stabilize or lower blood pressure, and bring a full round of oxygen to your body. In turn, this will cause you to relax and lower stress. I recently had an incident of feeling extremely lightheaded on a plane flight and automatically started slow deep breathing. Within a minute or two, I felt normal. Shallow chest breathing, on the other hand, limits the diaphragm's range of motion and can make you feel short of breath, lightheaded, and anxious.

How to engage in deep (diaphragmatic) breathing:

1. Lie down and place one hand (palm face down) on your chest and the other hand (palm face down) on your abdomen just below your ribcage.
2. Breathe normally and notice which hand is moving the most: the hand on the chest or the hand on the abdomen. Correct deep breathing means the abdomen will rise higher than the chest.
3. If not, try practicing this technique, a few times a day in any position, or in any place. Place your palms flat on your abdomen beneath your rib cage with your middle fingertips touching at a point two to three inches above your navel. Breathe in through your nose for a slow count to three and then exhale to the count of three.

ACUPUNCTURE

Acupuncture is an ancient Chinese medicine that involves inserting thin needles into specific points in the body for healing. We see mention of the practice in documents as early as 100 BCE.[14] Acupuncture remains only partially accepted within western medicine but is slowly becoming accepted as a viable alternative for those who prefer a drug-free option to treat disorders. Some medical insurance companies now cover acupuncture, but it's best to confirm what treatments are covered ahead of time.

TCM (Traditional Chinese Medicine) explains acupuncture as a way to balance the flow of energy known as qi or life force. Chinese medicine believes there are pathways called meridians where the energy flows through your body. If it is blocked or stagnant, illness can strike. The specific points that acupuncture needles are inserted into help rebalance the flow while removing illness and pain

Acupuncture is used to treat:

- Stress
- Stroke rehabilitation
- Headaches
- Asthma
- Many kinds of pain (dental, labor, back, neck)
- Osteoarthritis
- Sinus conditions
- Insomnia
- Anxiety and depression
- Digestive disorders

---

14   "brief history of acupuncture | Rheumatology | Oxford Academic." Accessed May 5, 2019. https://academic.oup.com/ rheumatology/article/43/5/662/1788282.

In contrast to traditional prescribed medicines, acupuncture results in few side effects. At times, a patient may experience slight bleeding or bruising at the site of needle insertion, but it is uncommon. As always, you should check with your primary doctor before starting acupuncture, or any, treatment. If needed, seek out a certified acupuncturist. Most states require specific certifications of practitioners before issuing a license.

Medical doctors are eligible to perform acupuncture if they have completed the required training. American Academy of Medical Acupuncture is the licensing organization for MDs. www.medicalacupuncture.org

I had weekly acupuncture treatment for three months as part of the overall program with Dr. Patton. I had no pain or issues with the needles and found it relaxing. As this was for a general condition (stress) and to boost immunity, I can't say definitively that it "cured" anything. However, I believe it did have positive benefits. I expected it to be a good experience since my oldest daughter had used acupuncture for migraine headaches for years with amazing results—even after many prescription medications did not help.

ENERGY WORK

....

> *Energy work is defined as techniques, originating from both ancient traditions and recent discoveries, used to manipulate the bioenergy of the patient with the goal of restoring harmony*

49

or removing blockages from within the body.
(Thefreedictionary.com)

Some believe that humans have, in addition to the 11 organ systems, separate energy systems or fields. Decades of research have led a number of doctors and alternative practitioners to believe there are multiple fields that serve different purposes in the human body. The conclusions range from three to nine energy systems that are responsible for healing the human body. While the traditional western medical community acknowledges the existence of an energy field in the body, namely the electromagnetic field (EM), it continues to be slow to embrace the multiple field concept. These beliefs are originally from many ancient traditions in various parts of the world. In the yogic traditions, it's called "prana." In Chinese traditions, it's called "qi" and incorporated in acupuncture, Tai Chi, and Qigong. In the Japanese Buddhist tradition, we see energy addressed in Reiki healing.

I asked Dr. Patton for recommendations on reading to learn more about the energy movement. I was experiencing a noticeable feeling of 'energy' that commenced shortly after the start of every acupuncture session and that soon transferred to my novice meditation sessions. My best description of the feeling was a low vibration that transmitted from my head to my toes. In response to my question on what this was Dr. Patton responded it was my "qi." He recommended Donna Eden's pioneering book *Energy Medicine*, written in 1998 expounding on her beliefs there are 9 separate energy systems in the body. I found it fascinating and now use many of the techniques in the book, including the daily warmup routine. Twenty years after the publication of Eden's book, energy medicine is coming to the forefront with scientific studies measuring the effectiveness of what can't be seen by the human eye. There are many additional books written on energy medicine now available from authors who have come to similar conclusions as Donna Eden.

RELAXATION TECHNIQUES

These can be done separately or in conjunction with meditation with the goal to increase your awareness of your body and refocus attention on something calming. Practicing regularly creates new neural pathways in your brain.

Muscle relaxation – Focus on slowly tensing and then relaxing each muscle group. You can start either in your toes and work up to your head or the reverse. Tense your muscles for about five seconds and then relax for 30 seconds, moving steadily up or down.

Visualization – This technique uses your imagination while you sit in a quiet spot. Close your eyes, if you wish. Loosen any tight clothing and concentrate on your breathing. Form mental images to take a visual journey to a peaceful, calming place such as the beach, the top of a mountain, or in the woods. Try and incorporate as many senses as you can, including smell, sight, sound and touch.

Other techniques include:

- Massage
- Biofeedback
- Aromatherapy
- Hydrotherapy

These techniques all have their attributes. If one does not work for you, try another. Be patient and do not let the process give you additional stress. An activity out there will work for you even if it's not one of these. Make sure to check the background and credentials of the company performing the technique.

Stress is not something that is going away in our modern world, and the ability to manage it will play an important role in living a long and vital life.

SPEND TIME IN NATURE

BEING IN NATURE (THE NATURAL OUTDOORS) used to be a normal part of daily living for those of us in the "older generation." As children, most of us lived in an environment where you were sent outside to play and told not to come back in for a good long while. No one checked where you were or what you were doing. Now, parents in most areas feel that outdoor play has to be scheduled and monitored.

Realizing my immune system had gone haywire and with no answers from the medical experts, I started to wonder how our environment and modern lifestyle might be affecting me. The research surprised me. The Consumer Product Safety Commission (CPSC) states:

> In the last several years, a growing body of scientific evidence has indicated that the air within homes and other buildings can be more seriously

polluted than the outdoor air in even the largest
and most industrialized cities. Other research in-
dicates that people spend approximately 90 per-
cent of their time indoors. Thus, for many people
the risk to health may be greater due to exposure
to air pollution indoors than outdoors.

Happily, a lack of being in nature wasn't on my list. By luck, divine guidance, or whatever source, I spend summers and fall right in the middle of nature, deep in the mountains of Colorado, which is a mecca of soaring peaks, lush forests, and rushing rivers and waterfalls. We open the windows for ventilation, and acres of woods, open fields and ascending peaks surround us. In the winter, while in a city environment, we live in a tropical and recreational area on the west coast of Florida with the beach five minutes away. We have the same ability to throw open the patio doors to the outside air, so we're lucky. The new terminology for the natural outdoors is green (grass and trees) and blue (water) spaces, and health experts plead with city planners to include these spaces in future city planning for health benefits for all ages. The concrete jungles and sealed environments that constitute our major cities have caused a need to schedule "time in nature."

Researchers in Philadelphia studied associations between urban restoration efforts and the mental health of its residents.[15] The study found that after "greening up" vacant

---

15   "Greening Vacant Lots Reduces Feelings of Depression in City
....." Accessed May 5, 2019. https://www.pennmedicine.org/news/
news-releases/2018/july/greening-vacant-lots-reduces-feelings-of-
depression-in-city-dwellers-penn-study-finds.

lots suffering from illegal dumping, overgrown vegetation and abandoned cars, the nearby residents expressed a 41% drop in depressive feelings and an almost 51% drop in feelings of worthlessness. The same study researched cleaned up vacant lots that did not have green restoration added. Those nearby residents did not experience the same reduction in negative mental health symptoms.

The concept to "green up" spaces has positive benefits to our health and is being studied in other urban areas such as Washington, D.C., Youngstown, Ohio, Flint, Michigan, and Camden, New Jersey. Its low cost and simple implementation could have a positive impact for people all over the US.

Being in nature promotes physical, mental and social health. The latest studies show a lower incidence of 15 diseases—including depression, anxiety, heart disease, diabetes, asthma and migraines—when spending a regular amount of time in nature. Being in nature reduces stress and drops blood pressure and heart rate. While scientists don't understand exactly why being in nature has the positive impact studies show, the results are enough for doctors and scientists to encourage everyone to make time for the outside in their schedules.

These two studies exemplify the impact of spending time in nature:

- A Vancouver 2015 study led by Jessica Finlay showed that spending time in nature is good for you on a physical, spiritual, and psychological level. The study concentrated on seniors aged 65-86 and showed that being in nature seemed to lower inflammation. Chronic Inflammation in the body can cause disorders and diseases.

- A 2016 study of 100,000 women conducted by the Environmental Health Perspectives, found no matter what age, socioeconomic status or race, people whose homes were surrounded by vegetation lived 12% longer. Within the 100,000 women in that study, there was a 34% lower rate of death from respiratory illness and a 13% lower rate of cancer death.

If you are not already incorporating "being in nature" into your schedule, please consider adding it in whether you visit a city park, beach, forest, mountains, or your own backyard garden.

THE MOUNTAINS

Living in a high-altitude mountainous regions provides health benefits, and studies show even short vacation visits can positively impact weight loss. Mountains may help you live longer and lower heart disease risk. Many of the top US counties for longevity were high-altitude counties in mountainous regions as reported in the Journal of the American Medical Association.

Mountains can provide health benefits that include: better sleep, easing of anxiety and depression, weight loss, and ease symptoms for asthma sufferers. Fresher air combined with an active outdoor lifestyle including hiking, mountain biking, skiing, snow shoeing, kayaking and others.

Olympic athletes train in high altitudes as it gives them an "edge" to their performance as extra blood vessels form in the heart to work more efficiently and adjust to a lower-oxygen environment. Most of us are not high performance athletes, Olympic or otherwise, but the statistics in these regions show lower rates of heart attack and stroke, and many lowered cancers rates as well for the general population. The average lifespan in the top three counties (all in high altitude Colorado) is 86 years while the average lifespan in US as of 2017 is 78.6 years according to the latest CDC mortality report.[16] As an aside, the average lifespan in the US has dropped by one tenth two years in a row, starting in 2015, a significant finding as these were the first drops in over 20 years across the general population. There is intense scrutiny to understand why. Theories include the ever-increasing obesity rate, the current opioid crisis, and possible environmental factors.

The mountains, especially at the highest peaks, have a high concentration of negative ions. Contrary to the description, a negative ion is of benefit to humans while positive ions are not. An ion is a charged atom or molecule. Negative ions have more electrons than protons. Positive ions have more protons than electrons and can turn into free radicals which can damage healthy cells and increase risk of disease. Nature has more negative ions in higher

_____

16   "Products–Data Briefs–Number 328–November 2018–CDC." 29 Nov. 2018, https://www.cdc.gov/nchs/products/databriefs/db328. htm. Accessed 6 May. 2019.

concentration. These ions are a mood booster and air purifier while offering the ability to kill bacterial organisms.

Our indoor sealed environments have limited amounts of negative ions, and indoor air conditioning usage makes it worse. While air conditioning makes us feel more comfortable, it creates less healthy air.

Testing shows an increased negative ion count after a thunderstorm that produces lightning. On mountain peaks, at the beach, and by waterfalls, negative ion count is also much higher, because sunlight, radiation, moving air or rushing water constantly break apart the molecules.

THE BEACH

Those beneficial negative ions in the mountains abound on the beach. The waves have negative ions which raise your mood, help alleviate depression, and promote a good night's sleep. Meanwhile, sea water can detoxify and function on an antibacterial level for your body just with your presence in the water. On a more cosmetic note, it can help with the elasticity of your skin without expensive creams or invasive treatments. Being in salt water has been shown to reduce symptoms for those who have rheumatoid arthritis, as well as improve many other conditions.

BENEFICIAL INGREDIENTS IN THE SEA:

MAGNESIUM:

Magnesium is needed for many functions in the body to perform well and helps with strong bones, balanced hormones, healthy nervous and cardiovascular system, and strong brain and heart functions. Sea water allows for a simple way to safely absorb magnesium through the skin.

POTASSIUM:

Potassium is one of the seven essential macrominerals to keep the body processes going. The proper amount of potassium provides enhanced muscle strength, regulates fluid balance, reduces the risk of stroke, lowers blood pressure, and preserves bone mineral density. Sea water is awash in it so to speak.

IODINE:

Your body absorbs the iodine in seawater, and the human body needs iodine to keep energy and metabolic levels running smoothly and hormone levels at proper levels. Iodine also has anti-carcinogenic properties and has been shown to reduce fibrocystic disease symptoms.

SEAWEED:

This food contains vitamins C and E, which help protect the skin from UV damage. It's a natural moisturizer and boosts natural collagen production. Its nutrients calm inflammation.

BROWN AND RED ALGAE:
This algae contains a compound called fucosterol, which decreases inflammation from the sun's rays and helps the body produce both collagen and antioxidant enzymes. The algae helps reinforce skin cell walls, so the cells retain moisture and block irritants.

SALT:
Let's not forget the salt in seawater. You certainly notice it if it gets in your eyes. Salt is detoxifying (think bath salts) and inhibits bacterial growth and skin infections.

FISH PROTEINS:
Amino acids and peptides derived from fish can help boost the production of collagen and strengthen hair and nails. These amino acids may help stave off wrinkles and sagging.

So jump and play in those waves, because you may be younger and healthier for it.

SAND:
Connecting with the Earth with bare feet is a primary source of "Earthing," which means grounding with the earth. I'll discuss that in some detail later. The beach is a perfect place to do this. As an extra benefit, wet sand acts as a natural exfoliant, which keeps skin clean, healthy and rejuvenated.

An odd fact I found in my research, as crazy as this sounds, is that a portion of the sand that we play and lay on is due to parrotfish poop. They excrete 840 lbs of eroded coral per year per large parrotfish to 11,000 lbs for the giant humphead parrotfish.

THE SUN

While considered something to worry about these days, sunshine is well known as our best source of vitamin D, an essential vitamin for our health. However, it has been confusing to know just what exposure you should have with unprotected skin versus when to wear sunscreen. Skin cancer rates are elevated these days, so caution is recommended. At the same time, a growing trend of dangerously low vitamin D levels has been found in our general population. We know that *some* level of sun exposure is helpful. Our skin will not absorb vitamin D with sunscreen applied, so most doctors recommend 15 minutes a day in the sun without sunscreen. Check with your doctor to have your levels checked if you don't know. You may be prescribed vitamin D supplements.

EARTHING

Earthing is a theory that our bodies are meant to come into direct contact with the Earth (a grounding force) to release positive ions, which are bad. The electromagnetic waves (EMF's) build up positive electrons, and we need to counteract this with negatively charged free electrons.

We have very little direct contact with the Earth these days. With high-rise buildings, elevated beds, and insulated shoes, we live in a space above the earth. Earthing theory says that walking outside barefoot and sitting, laying, or sleeping outdoors in direct contact with the earth provides health benefits.

A small number of scientific studies indicate Earthing provides benefits. A 2015 NIH study suggests that "grounding an organism produces measurable difference in the concentrations of white blood cells, cytokines, and other molecules involved in the inflammatory response." NIH also stated this about Earthing: "electrons from the Earth may in fact be the best antioxidants, with zero negative secondary effects, because our body evolved to use them over eons of physical contact with the ground."[17]

Some of the NIH study involving medical infrared imaging show inflammation levels decreasing from 30 minutes of connecting with the Earth. In addition, oxygen consumption and pulse and respiratory rates increased with an associated increase in blood oxygenation. While studies continue, the rest of us can be more mindful of taking the time to connect with the Earth in some way. It's an activity that costs us nothing.

Some of the possible benefits to following an Earthing protocol are:

- Improving sleep
- Improvement in body inflammation

---

17   "The effects of grounding (earthing) on inflammation, the ...–NCBI." 24 Mar. 2015, https://www.ncbi.nlm.nih.gov/pmc/articles/PMC4378297/. Accessed 6 May. 2019.

- Improvement in symptoms of autoimmune disorders
- Lowering stress levels
- Improving blood pressure
- Increased energy
- Releasing muscle tension and headache
- Rapid wound healing
- Anti-aging

This doesn't solve the difficulties if you live in winter climates or are not able to do this outside. You probably won't be surprised to learn that a whole range of products developed for indoor use can be purchased. If you do an online search, there are websites with products for Earthing. I can't vouch for the benefits of these products—I have never tried them—but it may be worth a web search to see what's available.

FOREST BATHING (SHINRIN-YOKU)

The Japanese government coined this term in the early 1980s and it basically means to spend time out in the woods. What we humans used to do naturally and without thought now has to be resurrected in modern times as a scheduled activity. While Japan took the lead in pouring money into research, which showed many health benefits to staying in the woods for a couple of hours—and even resulted in mandated forest bathing as a health benefit and funded walking paths in the forest across the country—the US is not far behind in promoting the activity. Forest bathing walks in nature parks and resorts in the US focus on immersion in nature. All the studies, whether in Japan or the US, indicate forest bathing lowers pulse rates and blood pressure, reduces the stress hormone cortisol, and boosts levels of immune-boosting human "natural killer" cells, which protect against viruses and cancers.[18]

When enough trees are cut down, it can affect rainfall, wind speed and the amount of pollution particles in the air in a particular area. While many countries are making a concerted effort to manage their forests sustainably, deforestation remains a huge problem for the earth. Trees themselves function by giving off oxygen which we humans must have, and are a key player in affecting climate change. Trees absorb carbon dioxide in enormous quantities (one of the greenhouse gases). Even nations who previously have ignored their severe pollution problems, such as China, are taking steps to improve their air. China has implemented a massive tree planting program near Beijing as a step to offset the severe air pollution there.

Try to incorporate activities in tree rich areas a few times a week, it could be a boost to your health. I walk in a park like atmosphere filled with trees in Florida and have a forest right outside my door in Colorado to explore when I'm there. For those who cannot get to these areas for whatever reason, gardening has been shown to have some of the same benefits. Even if you just grow plants in a few pots, you will bring the connection to nature into your life.

---

18   "Blood pressure-lowering effect of Shinrin-yoku (Forest bathing)–NCBI." 16 Aug. 2017, https://www.ncbi.nlm.nih.gov/pmc/articles/PMC5559777/. Accessed 10 May. 2019.

If you feel you would be better served by having someone guide you on a forest walk, there is now a national association called Nature & Forest Therapy (ANFT) which provides a certification program for Forest Therapy Guides. Check with their online site to search for a guide in your area. https://www.natureandforesttherapy.org

TAKE CARE OF YOUR BRAIN

I N MY QUEST TO FIND tools to help keep me in remission with my autoimmune disease, I realized that keeping the brain healthy was as crucial, if not more so, as keeping the body in general good health. I'm an avid reader, played piano as a child, took voice lessons as a teenager/young adult, and now am a watercolor painter, photographer, and writer. All of these activities have been found to have positive impact on the health of our brains while reducing the risk of developing dementia and keeping our intellect sharp. The latest research shows the brain's capabilities have been underestimated, and the newest findings could have a powerful effect on mental and physical health.

Harvard professor of psychology Ellen Langer, PhD, conducted a groundbreaking study in 1979, that is still frequently cited, which involved two groups of men in their 70s and 80s spending a week isolated with only 1950s memorabilia. One group was told to live as if they were young men in the 1950s while the second group was instructed to only *reminisce* about the 50s. Measurement tests were conducted before and after the tests. Afterward, dramatic changes appeared. Both groups were stronger and their joints more flexible. Height, weight, gait, posture, hearing, vision, and even IQ tests improved. The first group (who were living as if they were young men in the 50s) had significantly more improvement across the board than the second group (who were only reminiscing about the 50s). However, the reminiscing group still had an increase in positive changes. All this happened in *one week.*

From this, we learn that the mind/body connection is more impactful than previously known. Taking care of the brain appears to be a crucial component in living a long and healthy life. The aging process may not be the automatic road to wheelchairs, senility, and drooling in our food that we fear it is. Our mindsets may have a dramatic effect on how we age, and we can control our mindsets.

Newer studies of the brain indicate it is not the fixed and unchanging organ that it was thought for centuries. The brain can be trained. Mental abilities can be improved and damaged areas, as in a stroke, can possibly be rewired. Although I'm not a doctor or scientist, I think this means we have far more power individually to make positive changes to our health without medical intervention. Taking some responsibility into our own hands could mean the difference between a long vital life and the alternative: early physical and mental deterioration, which negatively affects our quality of life and possibly shortens it.

The scientists out there are finding that humans have complex interactions between the body's systems, which includes the immune system, that were previously unknown. Recent studies published in 2014 and 2018 associated with the National Center for Biotechnology Information and National Institute of Health suggest strong connections exist between the brain, gut, and immune systems. Until recently, brain and gut systems were thought to be totally separate entities. However, newer studies show complex interactions take place between these systems that impact the immune system. The gut microbiome (the microbes in your intestines) communicates with immune cells, which controls how your body responds to infection. In addition, the gut microbiome has millions of nerves that are connected to the brain and may affect brain health.

In this world of fast-moving medical discovery, it is worthwhile for everyone to try and stay abreast of the latest developments. Even as this book goes to print, I know more discoveries will be announced. If you develop health issues, one of these new fields may apply to you. You want a doctor who is up to date on the latest medical evolutions.

Some of the latest developmental fields:

- Neurogenesis – Researching the brain's ability to create new cells. Previously, it was believed the brain only had a finite number of cells in our lifetimes.

- Neurocardiology – Exploration of the heart's interaction and communication with the brain. Until recent years, the heart was believed to be an organ similar to many others, which functioned only with the brain's instructions.

- Neuroplasticity – The brain's ability to reorganize itself by forming new neural connections throughout life. Previously, the brain was thought to be static or hard-wired after childhood. This has far-reaching implications for stroke recovery, learning disabilities, and others.

- Gene Editing – The insertion, deletion, or replacement of DNA at a specific site in the genome of an organism or cell. This could be an answer to eliminating cancers and other genetic diseases.

- Neuroimmunology – A study of the nervous system and the immune system to develop treatments (immunotherapy) which use your body's own immune system to help fight cancers of many types.

DEMENTIA AND ALZHEIMER'S

For those of us marching toward the latter stage of life, we have more than a bit of anxiety wondering if these are in our future. **Alzheimer's is a progressive disease** of the brain that slowly causes impairment in memory and cognitive function. The exact cause is unknown and, as of now, no cure exists. Symptoms generally appear after age 65 but can appear as early as the 40s and 50s. Early-onset Alzheimer's is uncommon, affecting only 5% percent of the more than 5 million Americans with Alzheimer's. **Dementia is a syndrome—not a disease.** Dementia is a group of symptoms that affect mental cognitive tasks, such as memory and reasoning. Alzheimer's is a common cause of dementia. The latest figures from 2017 show an increase of 3.6% from the previous year to 5.7 million people who suffer from Alzheimer's and other dementias, which is expected to triple by 2050.[19]

As I get older, I wonder about maintaining my mental abilities. I find it distressing to read and hear about Alzheimer's and dementia waiting to strike the unsuspecting. It is a terrible fate for both the patient and the family. The latest research indicates there may be a genetic component to this disease. A gene variant called APOE is used as a "marker" of sorts. But simply because you or your family members have this does not mean you will have this condition.

Some good news: Research shows certain activities may help improve your memory and make you smarter. If you or a loved one has already been diagnosed with Alzheimer's or dementia, do not lose all hope. Music therapy is being used in over 4,500 facilities around the country to help memory, lower agitation and stress, and reduce the need for antipsychotic drugs in many Alzheimer's patients.

With all of the research being done, further advances in treatment may be just around the corner. Our baby boomer

19   "Alzheimer's Facts and Figures Report | Alzheimer's Association." https://www.alz.org/alzheimers-dementia/facts-figures. Accessed 6 May. 2019.

generation is so massive that it is driving movement and money to try and solve the problem of Alzheimer's and dementia.

Taking care of your brain can mean many things. First, include aerobic exercise, which benefits the brain no matter your age. Such exercise has been shown to boost nerve growth and improve the health of blood vessels. The earlier the better for brain-stimulating activities, and it can take the form of many different kinds of pursuits. I've listed some ideas below for you to consider.

Learn something new.

I have a near constant urge to learn about most any subject out there, which is increasing with age. Maybe this comes from a fear that I only have so much time left in this life, or maybe it's the realization that I have more to learn even as I learn more. Whatever the reason, I've been gratified to learn that this curiosity may help keep my brain younger and supple. Any new activity that is unfamiliar and mentally challenging provides social and mental stimulation. It may give you a new purpose in life and help take care of your brain in pursuit of a vital life.

Try online learning platforms on any subject that interests you.

They are for the most part free and offered by different prestigious schools and universities from around the world. Coursera, edX, Khan Academy, Alison, Udacity, Duolingo and others are available. Coursera is the largest of these platforms and the one I know best. I've taken a number of classes ranging from genetics to Roman architecture to literary fiction. Did I finish every class? No. Did I learn something from every class? Yes. Some were more compelling than others. Some were over my head in difficulty. In those cases, I felt relief in knowing there was no risk to me regarding dropping out.

Try your local college or university extended studies programs for in-person classes.

In some cases, your cost will be minimal if the college is promoting senior learning and your age qualifies you for such. They generally schedule classes at times convenient for most people.

Learn another language.

You've probably heard this one and wondered what was really behind it. In fact, there have been a number of studies done to show that learning another language stimulates and exercises the brain. Consistent exposure to the new language is more important than proficiency. A 2013 study at Northwestern University found bilingual speakers were better in their inhibitory control, which is the ability for someone to focus attention on one thing while tuning out extraneous outside interference.

Another study, conducted by Dr. Thomas Bak and his team from the University of Edinburgh in 2013, examined dementia factors in 648 dementia patients and found that bilingualism delayed the onset of dementia by 4.5 years on average. Education did not appear to affect the rate of onset and, in fact, bilingual *illiterate* patients experienced a delay in onset, too.

GAMES

A large number of computer brain fitness programs or "games" have been developed in the last few years and claim benefits, such as improved concentration, problem-solving, reaction time, and others. Neuroracer is one example of one of the more studied "brain" games out right now. It's a game developed by Dr. Adam Gazzaley of the University of California, San Francisco, which guides a car down a winding road while picking out flashing circles along the way. Their own studies, released in 2013, indicated significant cognitive improvement within the 60-85 year old group and they claim the effects lasted months after the game and study were done.

Newer independent studies show there appear to be some benefits from brain fitness games for older people who are at high risk of cognitive decline. However, the most positive results come from group activities with a trainer for brain training. Check with your local senior center for class availability. Whether there are equally positive benefits for at home online programs is unknown with initial independent research showing less than significant benefits. Some indication shows that, like all activities that are practiced frequently, improvement in skill and speed is likely but does not indicate increased cognitive abilities. Although there's little harm in participating in a computer fitness program, be aware that it should be used as part of an overall program of brain-enhancing activities.

CREATIVE ARTS

Drawing, painting, writing, playing musical instruments, singing, and other similar pursuits have been shown to stimulate creation of new neural connections in your brain. Creative arts, many research studies have confirmed, keep your brain young. With such a wide variety of choices within the "creative arts" category, everyone should be able to find at least one activity that fits their interest to incorporate in their life. Here are just a few:

Music

Music may help keep your brain young and supple according to all the latest research by stimulating and giving your brain a total workout. That includes playing *or* listening to music. You have an advantage if you ever had a minimum of 15 months of musical training in early life. The additional neural connections that were made could last a lifetime. This may be a defense against memory loss and cognitive decline in later years.

In a 2010 study, Harvard neurologist Catherine Wan and Gottfried Schlaug found music had a profound positive impact on the brain. The brains of adult professional musicians had a larger volume of gray and white matter that the brains of non-musicians.[20] White matter plays an im-

---

20   "Music Making as a Tool for Promoting Brain Plasticity across the Life …." https://www.ncbi.nlm.nih.gov/pmc/articles/ PMC2996135/. Accessed 7 May. 2019.

portant role in balance, walking, learning new things and the speed at which you learn. Gray matter involves learning skills and memory capabilities. Such findings speak to the brain's plasticity, the ability to change or adapt in response to experience, environment or behavior.

Researchers from Columbia University (2009) studied musicians versus non-musicians and found that musicians had an enhanced auditory system. This translated into an increased ability to identify pitch and detect and interpret other people's emotions. The complexity of music requires the brain to do a lot of work to make sense of it.

If you didn't have any musical training as a child, don't feel frustrated. You can start at any age. Studies indicate that older adults (ages 60 to 85) experienced significant gains in memory, verbal fluency, planning ability, and other cognitive functions after just six months of piano lessons. Studies also show merely listening to music can make a difference in both memory capabilities and cognitive functions. Try listening to different types of music, not just what you grew up with, because it challenges the brain. It has even been shown to reduce anxiety and improve mood and sleep quality.

Reading and Writing

Writing by hand may improve memory and increase skills that use the right and left brain. I read this with a bit of dismay, because my penmanship was never good. Over the years, my handwriting disintegrated to an almost illegible scrawl. I have not included this in my routine. As you can tell from this book, I'm concentrating on researching and writing down my story, and it's being done on a laptop. This, and other, types of writing stimulate the brain. You might start by writing down some lifetime memories or starting a journal.

A six-year study lead by Dr. Robert Wilson, senior neuro-psychologist at the Rush Alzheimer's Disease Center, reported findings that the lifetime readers and writers in a group of 294 elderly participants did better than others on their cognitive abilities. In addition, those participants showed no outward symptoms of Alzheimer's. However, when examined after death, there showed some evidence of the disease within their brains. (They had given prior permission for post-mortem testing). They were asymptomatic, a very important distinction.

This is not the only study released indicating it's possible to have evidence of Alzheimer's presenting in the brain without symptoms. It would seem that we might be able to impact the health of the brain with our choices in activities.

In other words, reading and writing on a regular basis could make a difference to your brain and how well it functions—even if your brain shows signs of dementia. Tests show that even if you didn't regularly read or write at a younger age, taking it up later in life may make a significant difference in cognitive decline. On the other hand, additional studies have shown that people who rarely read, write or do any activity that stretches their brain have a much higher than average rate of mental decline.

Reading books stimulates brain activity, and the effects remain several days after. This is about real reading, not skimming or just reading chapter titles and skipping to the end. Reading requires several different regions of the brain to work together making it a real workout for the brain. While reading any type of book on a regular basis appears to have a positive impact on the brain, research done at Stanford using an fMRI scanner showed different styles of reading had different levels of brain activity. Concentrated serious reading increased activity in more areas of the brain than pleasure reading.

Researchers at Yale University studied the records of 3,635 participants in the Health and Retirement Study on their reading habits. It was determined that people who read books regularly had a 20% lower risk of dying over the next 12 years compared with people who weren't readers or who read periodicals. The difference was the same regardless of race, education, state of health, wealth, marital status, and evidence of depression.

If you're not reading, start, or consider adding a writing project.

Art
A Mayo Clinic study tested people (middle age and older) engaging in artistic hobbies such as painting, drawing or sculpture and showed they were 73 percent less likely to develop mild cognitive impairment than those who didn't. Another study in Germany, (How Art Changes Your Brain: Differential Effects of Visual Art Production and Cognitive Art Evaluation on Functional Brain Connectivity July 1,

2014) compared brain scans of people who took painting and drawing classes with those who took art appreciation classes. The hands-on art class group showed the
most improved interaction between regions of the brain
associated with cognitive processes like introspection,
self-monitoring and memory. Creating art was more of a
total brain workout than simply observing.

In another study, Dr. Lora Likova, a scientist at Smith-
Kettlewell, transferred a drawing into raised-line images
for blind-from-birth individuals to learn how to draw.
Since the blind individuals could not see, their drawing
was from memory alone. After the week-long session in
which the individuals used their fingers to learn drawing,
fMRI brain scans showed increased activity of the visual
cortex in the brain, which is the area those of us with sight
use. The brain's ability to reorganize itself and adapt to
changing conditions in this way is called neuroplasticity.

FOOD SOURCES THAT SUPPORT
AND PROTECT THE BRAIN

Finally, don't forget to include foods that have been
shown to support the brain.

- Foods high in vitamin E: An antioxidant that protects the brain, which can be found in avocado, sun-
  flower seeds, beet greens, trout, butternut squash,
  swiss chard, safflower oil, wheat germ oil, peanuts,
  and peanut butter. Note: the most benefits found
  are from food, not vitamin E supplements.

- Red wine: Consuming moderate amounts may put you at reduced risk for Alzheimer's. One glass a day for women and two for men are the current recommendations from the US FDA.

- Fish: Even with concerns on pollution in our waters, the beneficial omega-3 fatty acids in fish can't be ignored. Salmon, mackerel, tuna, herring, and trout. Buy wild, if possible, for higher nutritional value.

- Foods high in B vitamins: Leafy greens, liver, eggs, legumes, chicken,turkey,pork, yogurt, and others all support brain health.

- Berries: These have antioxidants which may help stop age-related cognitive decline. Types with high levels include: blueberries, blackberries, cranberries, strawberries, acai berries, mulberries,black currents.

- Whole grains: Bulgar wheat, brown rice, barley, and oatmeal are all shown to lower risk of Alzheimer's.

- Eggs: Preferably organic, provides B-6, B-12, and choline, a micronutrient which is good for the brain.

- Dark chocolate: 70% or more cacao is a source of flavonoid (an antioxidant).

You can have a significant impact on the health of your brain by making relatively simple changes in your life, and these foods do not have the negative side effects prescription drugs do.

ALLEVIATING TOXICITY

Toxicity definition: the quality of being toxic or poisonous. (dictionary.com)

Toxic substances that cannot be eliminated from the body can cause disease, premature aging, and death.

TOXIC SUBSTANCES SURROUND US IN our environment— in our food and water, what we use on our bodies, the materials we put in our homes, and in our air. As I indicated in the introduction, toxicity is a major issue that has scientists concerned worldwide.

Don't make the mistake of thinking our government agencies have this under control. We are surrounded by chemicals every day – around 80,000 of them. They stem from the start of the Industrial Revolution, and the EPA is overwhelmed with the number. According to the EPA,

2,000 new chemicals are introduced each year, and the EPA is required to test them. A law passed in 2016 requiring more rigorous testing of chemicals has made an arduous system even more difficult. The EPA reviews a minimum of 20 chemicals at a time, and each has a seven-year deadline. The industry then has five years to comply with any requested new actions, such as reformulation. Decades could pass before getting through even the 1,000 most dangerous chemicals that the EPA has said needs urgent review.

Experts from NIH, Environmental Defense Fund, the World Health Organization, Project TENDR (a collaboration of leading scientists, health professionals and environmental and children's advocates) and others are raising alarm bells over what lasting effects all these chemicals may have on our bodies. Since the EPA doesn't have enough resources to test for everything except the most harmful of substances, we each need to take some action on our own and make changes in our own environments. My working theory is that my autoimmune disease manifested itself the minute my immune system had "topped" out on what it could handle, so I felt I needed to eliminate as much toxicity as possible. Further, I wanted to build up my immune system to withstand the inevitable attacks that would challenge me in the future. I didn't know which elements—activities, foods, stress, products I used (hair dye, makeup), the toxins in my carpet or paint, or something else—triggered it all.

Despite the staggering nature of this project, I felt determined to help myself as much as possible. Autoimmune disease cannot be cured, but it can enter indefinite re-mission. During my education process, I realized I didn't even understand *how* the human body expelled toxic substances much less the offenders (except in obvious well-publicized cases). I set myself the task to find out.

In "Principles of Toxicology," the NIH states that major routes for the elimination of chemical agents from the body are: from the kidneys to urine, from the liver to bile to feces, and from the lungs to exhaled air. To break it down:

- **Kidneys to urine:** The kidneys have to have ad-equate fluid to flush out toxins, which is their primary job.
- **Liver to bile to feces:** Your digestive system helps eliminate toxins. This means we need to eat a healthy diet and minimize stimulants and seda-tives, such as caffeine, alcohol, sleeping pills and other drugs.
- **Lungs to exhaled air:** The lungs take in oxygen and remove carbon dioxide with the inhalation and exhalation process. NIH states: With every breath, all of the airways except the mouth, and part of the nose, have special hairs, called cilia, that are coated with sticky mucus. The cilia trap germs and other foreign particles that enter your airways when you breath in air. These fine hairs then sweep the par-ticles up to the nose or mouth. From there they're swallowed, coughed, or sneezed out of the body. Nose hairs and saliva also trap particles and germs

The human body then spits, swallows, or expels it
out through a runny nose or a cough. [21]

According to scientists at NIH, the majority of cancers
are caused by environmental factors, which means not
genetic.[22] These factors include diet, lifestyle, pollution,
and exposure to toxins. This message varies from the one
I received years ago. Back then, the information leaned
strongly toward genetics as the most significant factor related to an individual's chances of developing cancer.

Currently, ongoing studies aim to determine if an increased risk of developing cancer or a secondary autoimmune disease occurs if you already have an autoimmune
disease. Even though no firm answers exist at this junc-
ture, the possibility motivates me to create a healthier environment for myself.

INDOOR ENVIRONMENT

Synthetic building materials, synthetic carpets, furni-
ture, fabrics and clothing, plastics, and urethane finishes
can emit benzene and formaldehyde. Trichloroethylene,
Xylene and Toluene are found in certain cleaners, paints,
polish, sealants, toner aids and are common in homes
and especially in office buildings. Office equipment, such

---

21   "How the Lungs Work | National Heart, Lung, and Blood
Institute (NHLBI)." 20 Nov. 2018, https://www.nhlbi.nih.gov/
health-topics/how-lungs-work. Accessed 10 May. 2019.
22   "Cancer is a preventable disease that requires major ...–NCBI-
NIH." https://www.ncbi.nlm.nih.gov/pmc/articles/PMC2515569/.
Accessed 8 May. 2019.

as copy machines, laser printers, and fluorescent lighting, can emit ozone. These factors, coupled with a "closed" environment where windows are mostly shut, could have negative health consequences. In addition, remember that air conditioning units deplete the air of negative ions, which are beneficial to us. The effects of indoor air pollutants range from minor, throat and eye irritation to more serious conditions such as respiratory disease and cancer.

OUTDOOR ENVIRONMENT

Air pollution is now the world's largest single environmental health risk, according to the World Health Organization. Of the 9 million deaths linked to pollution in 2015, 6.5 million were linked to air pollution, 1.8 million linked to water pollution, and one million linked to workplace pollution.

We *can* improve our individual home situation.

PLANTS

Add living plants in as many rooms as you can.

They are our friends and partners, and they take in carbon dioxide and other contaminants and enrich the air with oxygen. Plants emit water vapor that create a pumping action to pull contaminated air down around a plant's roots, where it is then converted into food for the plant. Thirty years ago, Bill Wolverton, the principal environmental scientist on the NASA Clean Air Study, released results on using plants to remove toxins from indoor air.

He published a book in 1997, entitled *How to Grow Fresh Air: 50 Houseplants that Purify your Home or Office*, for the general public based on his study. Even though the study is quite old, it is still considered the most definitive work to date. His book can still be purchased, and I personally own one. The findings were that certain plants were very effective in removing many of the common toxic substances found in homes. Top plants were palms, rubber tree, and dracaena on a sliding scale. The book has complete details on each of the 50 plants which were found to be the most effective in removing toxic chemicals from your indoor environment, including a rating scale, care instructions, and photos.

Kamal Meattle, CEO of Paharpur Business Centre in New Delhi, India found a unique solution to living and working in one of the world's smoggiest cities. After being told by doctors to move out of India due to the air pollution, he chose to stay and find a solution. He placed a plant-based air filtration system in his six-story office building. Air passes through his rooftop greenhouse of 400 plants. On top of that, he placed 800 plants throughout the offices and hallways. His top three plants are areca palm, mother-in-law's tongue, and the money plant. He did a TED talk on the subject in 2009 and has created systems for hundreds of homes in India's capital. People in other countries incorporate plants, as well. Japan is putting ecological gardens in hospitals. In Brazil, plants are used in mercury-contaminated gold trade shops to absorb the chemical. In China, where an estimated one million die from air pollution every year, a plan to plant trees was implemented to combat the problem. They've planted

32,400 square miles of them, employing 60,000 soldiers to do the work.

HIMALAYAN SALT LAMPS

These attractive lamps consist of a block of Himalayan salt with a small bulb inside that can generate negative ions. It's not a substitute for being in nature, because the amounts generated remain small. However, I find it worthwhile to add as a counter to unhealthy substances. Salt lamps attract mold, bacteria, and allergens to their surface due to their hygroscopic (water is attracted to its surface and then evaporates quickly) nature. They can possibly reduce allergy and asthma symptoms.

For better sleep, use the lamps with their yellow orange glow at a low setting. These can be good for people with seasonal light disorder and can boost moods. One pound of salt will filter approximately a 4x4 area, so buy multiple small lamps or larger sizes. Make sure the lamp is 100% Himalayan salt, because cheaper alternatives do not work in the same way. Since the heat interaction with the salt is what makes it effective, the lamp must produce heat. You may have noticed these lamps are suddenly for sale everywhere—even in drugstores. Himalayan salt is only found in the mines of Khewra, Pakistan in the western part of the Himalayan mountains, so make sure the label of origin is from Pakistan.

If you are worried about not being ecological, it's esti-mated at the rate of current mining, the salt supply should last at least another 350 years. The wood base is generally a sustainable wood called neem and the low wattage bulb consumes little energy.

HAND AND LIQUID SOAPS, FOAM AND GEL SOAPS, AND BODY WASHES

Avoid antibacterial unless you're sure it is reformulated.

Having read early studies on the negative effects of antibacterial products, I avoided them for years. For many people, "antibacterial" seemed the correct direction to take when purchasing soap products. As it turns out, the FDA found unsafe ingredients and issued a ruling that manufacturers have to remove the ingredients and reformulate their products within a year. The deadline was July 2017, but it is unknown how long the turnover will take in stores. Reading the labels for reformulated language is another task for the consumer.

The problems with the products were:

- Ingredients were not proven to be safe long term.
- Ingredients were not proven to be any more effective than regular soap and water.

These ingredients have been linked to helping cause antibacterial resistant germs which has been an ever growing problem. Nineteen ingredients have been removed with three remaining—benzalkonium chloride, benzethonium chloride and chloroxylenol. The FDA requires that manufacturers submit new safety and effectiveness data on those. Even with the new formulations, I would proceed with caution on any of these products. The government takes a long time to make changes for our safety when it comes to products that we use.

The FDA has asked for additional data from manufacturers to show that active ingredients are generally recognized as safe and effective. However, the government has not issued a mandate to recall these products.

Washing your hands with water alone can take 40 to 50% of the bacteria off without soap. Vigorous hands rubbing together under the faucet for at least 10 seconds is called for. If you're in a place with no regular soap or with antibacterial soaps of unknown origin, have some comfort in knowing what some doctors have known for a while—water will do a decent job and is much better than doing nothing.

HOME CLEANING PRODUCTS

For your home cleaning, there are enough choices to make your head spin and enough chemical ingredients to alarm you. Multiple cleaning products for different surfaces in the same room remains a common problem. As an example, you probably use a toilet bowl cleaner, a cleaner for the toilet surface, another cleaner for the shower, and then a glass cleaner for a shower door. If you're doing this at the same time, which most people do, it means you're exposing yourself to a new—and not improved—chemical compound in the air that comes from mixing chemicals. In doing research for this section, I first thought about how I had changed so many cleaning products to safer ones in my own home. However, I realized that I hadn't altered nearly the amount I thought I had and even the "green" products flooding the market now are not held to similar standards as are our food or medicines by the FDA. [23]

Experts present conflicting opinions. Tom Natan, a chemical engineer with the non-profit National Environmental Trust, says cleaning products available should be safe in small amounts and with proper ventilation.[24] but a recent NIH study suggest increased likelihood of developing symptoms such as headaches, asthma attacks, rashes, and even seizures.[25] You can go the route of severity and throw out all your commercial cleaners and make your own with a combination of white vinegar, washing soda, and baking soda. For me, I know I won't go to that extreme. Instead, my approach is to use a combination of natural ingredients when it makes sense, doing enough research to pick a "safer" cleaner, and ceasing the use of multiple cleaners in the same cleaning session.

23 "Cleaning Supplies and Household Chemicals | American Lung ...." https://www.lung.org/our-initiatives/healthy-air/indoor/indoor-air-pollutants/cleaning-supplies-household-chem.html. Accessed 8 May. 2019.
24 "The Truth About 'Green' Cleaning Products-Live Science." 6 Aug. 2007, https://www.livescience.com/1737-truth-green-cleaning-products.html. Accessed 8 May. 2019.
25 "Cleaning at Home and at Work in Relation to Lung Function Decline ...." 1 May. 2018, https://www.ncbi.nlm.nih.gov/pubmed/29451393. Accessed 8 May. 2019.

You can look at research that EWG (Environmental Working Group) does. They are a 25-year-old nonprofit organization that specializes in research and advocacy in the areas of toxic chemicals, public lands, agricultural subsidies, and corporate accountability. EWG researches more than 2,000 cleaning products, yet they are not without their share of controversy. EWG has been accused of biased ratings of products from companies owned by various members on their board of directors. Once again, I follow a common sense approach for me. I review ratings yet maintain skepticism for anything that doesn't ring true. I'm currently using both Method and Mrs. Meyer's products as I have some comfort with their ingredients. I still use various "traditional" cleaners and probably won't eliminate them altogether.

Note: Let's not forget that all of our cleaners end up down the drain and, ultimately, end up in our rivers and other bodies of water. Responsible usage is called for.

FLOOR COVERINGS

Unless we're starting from scratch in our home environment, there's a limit to what we can or will do to eliminate the toxins inside. Flooring is a more difficult issue to resolve than changing soaps and cleaners. Wall to wall carpet should be avoided by people with asthma or allergies as the nature of the product means it collects dirt, dust, and dust mites. In addition carpet has chemicals called VOCs (volatile organic compounds). The EPA states that VOCs in carpeting release gases into the air. Immediate symptoms can range from eye, nose, throat irritation to dizziness, fatigue and headaches, according to the CDC (Centers for Disease Control). The EPA states health effects may cause damage to the liver, the kidneys and the central nervous system. Some studies show these gases have caused cancer in animals, and some are suspected to cause cancer in humans. The EPA also states the gases are released in the highest amounts right after carpeting is installed, falling to low levels 48-72 hours after installation with proper ventilation.

The carpet and rug industry has a voluntary testing program (CRI-Carpet and Rug Institute), in place since 1992, that's meant to reduce emissions. In addition, CRI has certifications for low level VOC emissions through their program Green Label Plus (GLP), which is their voluntary indoor air quality testing program. Since its inception, the GLP program has had significant impact on the reduction of formaldehyde, which is one of the gases released. Ask your local carpet store for their low VOC or "green" carpet choices. You'll be buying a product better for your health. Keep in mind, this does not address any other chemicals and compounds beyond VOCs and may not address chemicals in the backing fabric, padding, or stain resistant treatments. I will be replacing carpet soon and plan on staying elsewhere for two nights after the installation even though I am buying a "green" low VOC product.

As with all products, the consumer should be wary of the marketing lingo. "Sustainable," "eco-friendly," and "recycled" sound great but don't actually mean healthier or safer. And carpeting should not be put in damp areas, as the effects of VOCs, dust, dirt, and dust mites are exacerbated.

Safer flooring choices include:

- **Ceramic tile:** Made of clay or other natural minerals and zero VOC's.
- **Hardwood flooring:** This should not be confused with laminate flooring, a synthetic product which may contain high levels of formaldehyde.
- **Linoleum flooring:** Linoleum is made from all-natural and biodegradable materials including linseed oil, cork, dust, pine resin, and wood flour.

Vinyl flooring, which is considered to be quite toxic, is made with many possibly unsafe products, including phthalates. Some national retailers (Home Depot, Menards, Lowe's, and Lumber Liquidators) have taken steps to remove phthalates from their vinyl flooring, which should be indicated on the labels.

RUGS

The market has been flooded with low-cost synthetics in the last few years, and they have possible emissions of their own, which could contribute to your indoor air pollution. Other options on the market vary in cost. Depending on the choice, the cost increase may be substantial. The benefit here is better possible air quality, and some of these materials last many, many years.

Healthier rug options

- Jute
- Wool
- Organic cotton
- Seagrass
- Sisal
- Coir

Jute, in particular, will be lower in cost, because it does not require pesticides or fertilizers to grow. Make sure to look for non-toxic backing that is sewn on—not glued.

PAINT

Paint also can contain VOCs. Older paints can continue to release low-level toxic emissions into the air for years. These days, many brands of low to zero VOC paints are available. This will be marked on the label.

PERSONAL CARE PRODUCTS

Unfortunately, the government has limited oversight over personal care products. These products include but are not limited to: shampoos, perfumes, makeup, deodorants, moisturizers, fingernail polishes, and hair dyes. The only government oversight of these products is the Federal Food, Drug, and Cosmetic Act, which passed in 1938 and focuses mainly on misbranding or false packaging. Premarket safety assessments, mandatory registration, and government ingredient review is not required in the US as it is in other countries. Further, the FDA does not have the ability to recall a product. There has been recent legislation under consideration in Congress (Personal Care Product Safety Act) to rectify this but, as of this publishing, it has not passed. The nature of most personal care products means they are being applied to your skin and absorbed. Experts recommend looking for products free of phthalates, parabens, and retinyl palmitate. There is an increase in companies producing products using organic materials that should be under consideration as well.

ELIMINATING TOXINS ALREADY IN THE BODY

Researchers say there are a few things you can incorporate in your life to help your body eliminate the toxins even though it's virtually impossible to eliminate all of the sources.

- Eat organic as much as possible for reduction of various pesticides and antibiotics.
- Exercise to help flush chemicals from the body.
- Cutting down on saturated fat may help. (Fat provides a place for toxins to remain in the body.)
- Open your windows for cleaner air unless you live in a city with heavily polluted air.
- Replace plastic with glass for food storage. Chemicals from the plastic can leach into food, especially when heating the plastic.
- Drink water, which can flush toxins from the body.

You may be surprised that sweating, i.e. using a sauna, is not listed here. Initial research showed promising information on the detox qualities of saunas, but they were alternative sources and not reputable health sites such as the NIH, Harvard, or Mayo Clinic, etc. In fact, expert after expert insisted that only the liver, intestines, and kidneys, along with the immune system, have the capability of removing toxins from the body. The jury is still out on the benefit of saunas and, in particular, infrared saunas. As for cleanses and colonics, there should be no need to use any of these products. Experts at NIH do not recommend these products under any circumstance and warn that some of the products and procedures could be harmful to your health.[26]

Many doctors and scientists believe we are an overprescribed nation. Certainly, medications deserve their place in the correctly prescribed dosage for specific treatments. Situations have arisen, such as with overprescribed antibiotics, in which resulting outbreaks of antibiotic-resistant "superbugs" create difficulties in treating some illnesses. Additionally, an administered drug dose can be toxic in one person, therapeutic for another and have no effect for a third. You might find it helpful, and even lifesaving, to work with a physician knowledgeable on these issues.

Our world is filled with substances that didn't exist in prior times. We should educate ourselves and understand how the makeup of our individual environments may affect us and adjust or eliminate as many potentially harmful substances as possible for healthier living.

26   ""Detoxes" and "Cleanses" | NCCIH." 24 Sep. 2017, https://nc-cih.nih.gov/health/detoxes-cleanses. Accessed 9 May. 2019.

HAVE A PURPOSE IN LIFE

THIS TOPIC IS A BIT more ethereal than previous chapters, and I purposely left it until last for that reason. Throughout this book, I've discussed concrete steps you can take to support and protect your body to live a longer and healthier life. Yet internal, soul-searching changes that touch you to your core turn out to be as important, or more so, than the rest. People who understand and maintain a conviction about why they're on this earth—and know what gives deep meaning to their lives—are much more likely to live longer and be healthier than those who don't.

What is your purpose in life?

If I had been asked prior to my autoimmune diagnosis, I could have answered easily and without thought. After the diagnosis, I felt unsure and off balance. Part of those feelings stemmed from feeling that I had no control over my situation and could not get satisfactory answers about my health. The stripping away of superficialities—just like the falling out of all my hair—exposed the bare truth that I no longer knew myself, my core self, nor was certain what gave my life deep meaning.

We define a purpose as your goals or aims in life—or whatever gives deep meaning to you. For some people, this can be connected to a vocation or volunteer work. For others, it can be expressed through their religious or spiritual beliefs or family. Motivation and responsibility lives behind whatever gives you deep meaning, and you will not easily find a true purpose in life if it is spent in self-absorbed and ego-driven actions. For most, a purpose in life will change over a lifetime as we grow and change. The entire process involves being open and listening to your own inner voice rather than the voices of others. Studies show that having a purpose in life appears to be just as important as the grounded day-to-day practices, such as food decisions and exercise routines, for your health and vitality. Having a purpose in life is linked to a longer life, a lowered risk of diseases, better sleep, and even a delay of the inevitable physical decline as we age. [27]

What did this have to do with my own journey through the autoimmune morass? The messages from different sources indicate that the mind and body connection is much stronger than previously thought and could have positive implications for our wellness and longevity. This

---

27   "Is purpose in life associated with less sleep disturbance in older adults ...." 10 Jul. 2017, https://sleep.biomedcentral.com/articles/10.1186/s41606-017-0015-6. Accessed 9 May. 2019.

gave me pause. What if it were possible to make a difference in my health and in my immune system by what I thought and believed? Could I make an impact to my health by the practices I kept and the faith/beliefs that I maintained? Depending upon your thought process, this is either a broad or narrow subject.

- Do you go through your days aimlessly or have goals for the future?
- Do you work in a job that you despise or do you feel fulfilled in your career path?
- Do you have hobbies which you participate in regularly?
- Do you practice mindfulness or rush through your days?
- Do you participate in programs that help others or avoid them?

A sense of purpose does not have to be a larger-than-life project which takes precedence over everything else. Smaller goals such as volunteering your time to connect and help other people can go a long way to helping answer the question about what gives you meaning in your life.

Let me clarify that I'm not talking about happiness when I reference "purpose." Happiness and life purpose are not the same. A purpose-driven life may ultimately increase happiness but not necessarily. Happiness is a fleeting state which comes and goes at a whim. The chase to find it ultimately ends in dissatisfaction for many. Having deep meaning in your life will provide strength and a sense of fulfillment that transcends the negative influences that come and go in our lives. Our purpose reflects our self, which is the unique soul in every individual.

Aristotle said in *Nicomachean Ethics* (written around 340BC) that a life of gratification (pleasure, comfort) and a life of money-making is a far lesser happiness than a virtuous life. What was true then holds true now. So how to find this magic purpose in life? At this point, I'm fairly certain I'm not going to be the person who discovers the cure for cancer. My own purpose in life now seems to be about being part of something bigger and passing on what I've learned about our minds and bodies.

An individual transformation can happen at any time. If you're unsure about what might give true meaning to your life, you could start by reflecting on those urges and interests that you may have wanted to start yet never did. Maybe the timing wasn't right or you pushed those thoughts away as unimportant. Take a chance and realize that you are the only one who can decide what's important to you.

My mind/body decided to let me know in no uncertain terms that I needed to stop and review what I was doing. The internal changes for me have been profound and led me to some interesting revelations:

- I realized that we make a choice with every action, thought and deed on how we perceive ourselves and others.
- I discovered that I cared far less about what other people thought than about making a difference and

acting with grace. By that, I mean leave fears and emotions out of a decision, have empathy and consider the long-term impact my decisions.

- My inner self was the real essence of me—not the outer physical self—and I needed to learn everything I could about that self and rely on my inner convictions and intuition when making changes.

- I believe that we are truly all connected and even a small action alters a course and direction for more than me. I find myself acting with ever increasing altruistic behavior without forethought.

- I have a growing conviction that my purpose in life might possibly be to continue to learn about myself and the world around me and pass on that knowledge.

STAY CONNECTED AND HELP OTHERS

In the journey to better health and a longer life, it appears part of the equation is not acting as if you live on a desert island. The modern world and all of its technology, which allows us to function fully without touching or speaking to another human face to face, is not good for us. Many scientists, including US surgeon general Vivek H. Murthy and Rob Reich, professor of political science at Stanford University, reference the negative mental and physical effects that are recognized from this isolation. Staying connected and helping others while giving back is a good way to combat this.

It's scientifically proven that giving back and helping others makes us feel happier and more content. It could be the start of a path to finding deeper meaning in your life. Endless organizations in our communities need our help and would welcome our involvement. Find your own path of interest and connect with others as a volunteer. Doing so strengthens social bonds and will enrich your life. The gift of your time and connection, rather than just money, can infuse your life with deeper meaning.

Connecting regularly with people combats loneliness and depression and puts us squarely back in the middle of our social world. Joining a volunteer organization or even starting a non-profit allows us to be in the center of connection with humanity. Isolation in the modern world is increasingly pointed to as a contributing factor in depression, mental illness, a reduced life span, and physical illnesses. Incorporate meaningful connection with other people in your life—not just texting or communicating via social media.

FAITH

Faith is wrapped around an individual's purpose in life so tightly that it almost can't be untangled. Faith means different things to different people.

Faith is defined as: *Firm belief in something for which there is no proof or something that is believed especially with strong conviction.* (Merriam-Webster.com)

Recent studies show that faith is a strong part of living a long vital life. Researchers have found that faith of any kind, a belief system in which people regularly incorporate in their lives, helps people live longer. Some type of faith or belief system appears to positively affect your health, which can be either of a religious or spiritual nature. How exactly this works is somewhat of a mystery.

The terms "spiritual" and "religious" used to be indistinguishable yet modern times have changed that. You can be spiritual without being religious, and religious without being spiritual. The following are a few examples of definitions as there are many interpretations.

- Religion: *A broad concept with multiple meanings. A system of beliefs and practices illustrating a code of morality and humanity's place in the world. The belief in a god or in a group of gods, an organized system of beliefs, ceremonies, and rules used to worship a god or a group of gods.* Vocabulary.com
- Religious: *Besides meaning "having to do with religion," it can mean relating to or manifesting faithful devotion to an acknowledged ultimate reality or deity.* Merriam-Webster.com
- Spirituality: *The quality of being concerned with the human spirit or soul as opposed to material or physical things.* oxforddictionaries.com

A study involving 4,000 people ages 64-101 in North Carolina, which was published in the Journal of Gerontology: Medical Sciences, showed people who attended religious services once a week were less likely to die in a given time period—even after eliminating control factors such as age, race, how sick they were among others. In this study, the percentage of people living longer who attended religious services once a week was equated to that of people who don't smoke over those who do, which showed a dramatic difference.

Thousands of research studies have been done on the association between what is designated R/S (Religion/Spirituality) and Health between 2000 and 2012 according to Harold G. Koenig, a psychiatrist at Duke University. His study, which analyzed many of those studies, found R/S had significant positive impact on many aspects of mental and physical health over those that had no spiritual or religious beliefs.

Other research studies done with people who had deeply held spiritual beliefs but no associated religious beliefs, compared with those who had no prescribed beliefs (spiritual or religious) showed better health results in the group holding spiritual beliefs. The spiritual group experienced lower levels of depression, anxiety and better health with fewer strokes.

Following a traditional religious practice or your own spiritual beliefs helps with the search for personal meaning, but how high people place that practice or belief in importance is dependent on a host of criteria including age, geographic location, race and ethnicity, income, education, and political affiliation, according to a Pew research study entitled, "Where Americans Find Meaning in Life."

With the deep inward reflection of the last few years, I have developed an intense interest in studying the world's major religions and other spiritual and alternative teachings.

This could possibly take the rest of my life given the immensity of the project. I've become aware there is a lot out there that's not explainable in our literal and physical senses world. As I mentioned before, meditation brought on odd sensations, visions almost, that happened with enough regularity to have me question my beliefs. I've become highly sensitive to nature, meaning I sense energy in things I wasn't aware had any—trees, plants and bond with wild creatures.

Even though I was brought up under traditional religious tenets, I remain unconvinced that attending worship in a physical building called a church, synagogue, temple, mosque, or other—led by a man or woman trained in whatever religious teachings of that particular sect—can bring me closer to God or the divine. I am painstakingly creating a whole belief system piece by piece that is uniquely mine. For me, this journey is an ongoing process wrapped up into my purpose in life. The process involves more searching, learning and absorbing to help me make some sense of my world and my place in it. I suspect it's the same urge that has brought people together for many centuries—how to incorporate our experiences and beliefs into our lives. We can find commonalities of core beliefs in all the major world religions. As the earth's people, we are more together than apart even if the world feels divided in these times.

While the search for life's meaning and the essence of oneself is a solitary process, it can send you in the direction of connection with other like-minded individuals. I was gratified to find company in this strange and wonderful process. Whether prompted by a traumatic event, a mid-life crisis, an illness, or perhaps just a strong desire to know or learn more about the self, other people are on the path to find purpose.

As of this writing, I am in a three-year remission without any sure way to know what, if anything, I've done to maintain a healthier body, mind, and soul has made a difference. What I do believe is that all these pieces have had a profound impact on my life, wellness, and satisfaction. Perhaps that's enough.

ADDITIONAL READING

Cave, James. "Hawaii's White Sand Beaches Are Made From Parrotfish Poop." March 29, 2014. https://www.huffpost.com

Congress–S.726 Personal Care Products Safety Act. March, 7, 2019. https://www.congress.gov

Duncan, David Ewing. "Chemicals Within Us." October 2006. https://www.nationalgeographic.com

FAO Food and Agriculture Organization of the United Nations. "The State of the World's Forests." 2018 https://www.fao.org

Langer, Ellen. "Science of Mindlessness and Mindfulness." November 2, 2017. https://www.onbeing.org

Perkins, Judy. "I'm the Woman Whose Terminal Breast Cancer Went Into Remission After Immunotherapy." June 6, 2018. https://www.womenshealthmag.com

Stamets, Paul. "6 ways mushrooms can save the world." June 11, 2008. https://www.TED.com

Sweet, Joni. "Experts Throw Cold Water on Study that Recommended No Alcohol." August 29, 2018. https://www.healthline.com

Vidyasagar, Aparna."What is CRISPR?" April 20, 2018. https://www.livescience.com

Watson, Elaine. "Do consumers expect kombucha to contain live organisms?" August 21, 2018. https://www.foodnavigator-usa-com

RESOURCES BY CHAPTER

Please note I chose to modify reference style by alphabetized references within each chapter and article published date rather than access date.

INTRODUCTION

American Heart Association. "Heart Disease and Stroke Statistics-2019 Update: A Report from the American Heart Association." January 2019. https://www.ahajournals.org

Gupta, Ruchi. "Almost half of food allergies in adults appear in adulthood." October 27, 2017. https://www.acaai.org

Levine, Hagai. et al. "Temporal trends in sperm count: a systematic review and meta-regression analysis." July 25, 2017. https://www.academic.oup.com

National Health Statistics Reports. "State Variation in Meeting the 2008 Federal Guidelines for Both Aerobic and Muscle-strengthening Activities Through Leisure-time Physical Activity Among Adults Aged 18-64: United States, 2010-2015." June 28, 2018. https://www.cdc.gov

Nuwer, Rachel. "What Happens When Western and Traditional Chinese Medicine Merge." Nov. 5, 2014. https://www.smithsonianmag.com

Rattue, Grace. "Autoimmune Disease Rates Increasing." June 22, 2012. https://www.medicalnewstoday.com

Shah, Amy. "Why Allergies & Autoimmune Diseases Are Skyrocketing." 2015. https://www.mindbodygreen.com

Wong, Shirley S. "A Push to Back Traditional Chinese Medicine With More Data." Nov 3, 2014. https://www.wsj.com

CHAPTER 1—KEEP PHYSICALLY ACTIVE

Abrahin, Odilon, et al. "Swimming and cycling do not cause positive effect on bone mineral density: a systematic review." July-August 2016. https://www.sciencedirect.com

American Journal of Health Promotion. "Effect of Two Jumping Programs on Hip Bone Mineral Density in Premenopausal Women: A Randomized Controlled Trial." January 1, 2015. https://www.journals.sagepub.com

Andersen, Oddbjorn, et al. "Bone Health in elite Norwegian endurance cyclists and runners: A cross-sectional study." 2018. https://www.bmjopensem.bmj.com

Arthritis Foundation. "12 Benefits of Walking." https://www.arthritis.org

Caspersen, C.J., Powell, K.E., Christenson, G.M. "Physical activity, exercise, and physical fitness: Definitions and distinctions for health-related research." March 1985. https://www.ncbi.nim.nih.gov

Donovan, Michelle. "Pumping iron: Lighter weights just as effective as heavier weights to gain muscle, build strength." July 12, 2016. https://www.brighterworld.mcmaster.ca

Journal of Sport and Health Science. "The effects of Tai Chi exercise on cognitive function in older adults: A meta-analysis." December 2013. https://www.sciencedirect.com

Loughborough University. "Hopping could reduce fracture risk for older people." September 10, 2015. https://www.iboro.ac.uk

NCCIH -National Center for Complementary and Integrative Health. "Yoga: In Depth." October 2018. https://www.nccih.nih.gov

NCCIH- National Center for Complementary and Integrative Health. "National Health Interview Survey 2017." November 2018. https://www.nccih.nih.gov

Nellis, Bob. "Mayo Clinic discovers high-intensity aerobic training can reverse aging processes in adults." March 10, 2017. https://www.newsnetwork.mayoclinic.org

Quinn, Elizabeth. "The important Link Between Exercise and Healthy Bones." June 6, 2018. https://www.nmortho.com

Robinson, Matthew M., et al. "Enhanced Protein Translation Underlies Improved Metabolic and Physical Adaptations to Different Exercise Training Modes in Young and Old Humans." March 7, 2017. https://www.cell.com

Rubin, Courtney. "The Benefits of Walking." January 6, 2015. https://www.realsimple.com

Sagon, Candy. "Lifting Lighter Weights As Effective As Heavy Ones." October 31, 2016. https://www.aarp.org

U.S. Department of Health & Human Services, Office of Disease Prevention and Health Promotion. "Physical Activity Guidelines for Americans." 2018. https://www/health.gov

CHAPTER 2—EAT HEALTHY BALANCED DIET

Annals of Internal Medicine. "Enough is Enough: Stop Wasting Money on Vitamin and Mineral Supplements." December 13, 2013. https://www.annals.org

Baudry, Julia, et al. "Association of Frequency of Organic Food Consumption with Cancer Risk." December 2018. https://www.jamanetwork.com

Burton, Robyn, Sheron, Nick. "No level of alcohol consumption improves health." August 23, 2018. https://www.thelancet.com

EUFIC (European Food Information Council).. "Mediterranean style diet might slow down aging, reduce bone loss." May, 2016 https://www.sciencedaily.com

FDA – United States Food & Drug Administration. "Dietary Supplements." https://www.fda.gov

Geller, Andrew, et al. "Emergency Department Visits for Adverse Events Related to Dietary Supplements." October 15, 2015. https://www.nejm.org

Harvard Health Publishing. August 22, 2018. " Health benefits of taking probiotics." https://www.health.harvard.edu

Hu, Zhihua, et al. "Bottled Water: United States Consumers and Their Perceptions of Water Quality." February 21, 2011. https://www.ncbi.nlm.nih.gov

Luciano, Michelle, et al. "Mediterranean-type diet and brain structural change from 73 to 76 years in a Scottish cohort." January 31, 2017. https://www.ncbi.nim.nih.gov

McEvoy, Miles. "Organic 101: What the USDA Organic Label Means." March 22, 2012. https://www.usda.gov

McIntosh, James. "Fifteen benefits of drinking water." July 16, 2018. https://www.medicalnewstoday.com

Popkin, Barry, et al. "Water, Hydration, and Health." August 2010. https://www.ncbi.nim.nih.gov

Postman, Andrew. "The Truth About Tap." January 5, 2016. https://www.nrdc.org

USDA -United States Department of Agriculture. "Organic Standards." https://www.ams.usda.gov

USPSTF-United States Preventive Service Task Force. "Vitamin Supplementation to Prevent Cancer and CVD: Preventive Medication." February 2014. https://www.uspreventiveservicetaskforce.org

CHAPTER 3—MANAGE STRESS

Azuma, K, et al. "Chronic Psychological Distress as a Risk Factor for Osteoporosis." December 1, 2015. https://www.ncbi.nlm.nih.gov

Eden, Donna. 2008 *Energy Medicine*. New York: Penguin Group.

Future Science OA . "The effects of chronic stress on health: new insights into the molecular mechanisms of brain-body communication." November 2015. https://www.ncbi.nlm.nih.gov

Hoge, Elizabeth, et al. "Loving-Kindness Meditation practice associated with longer telomeres in women." April 2013. https://www.sciencedirect.com

Holzel, Britta, et al. "Mindfulness practice leads to increases in regional brain gray matter density." 2010. https://www.sciencedirect.com

Luders, Eileen, et al. "The unique brain anatomy of meditation practitioners: alterations in cortical gyrification." February 29, 2012. https://www.frontiersin.org

Luders, Eileen, et al. "Forever Young(er): potential age-defying effects of long-term meditation on gray matter atrophy." https://www.frontiersin.org

MGH-Massachusetts General Hospital. "Mindfulness meditation training changes brain structure in 8 weeks." January 21, 2011. https://www.massgeneral.org

NIH- National Center for Complementary and Integrative Health. "Acupuncture: In Depth." Last updated: January 2016. https://www.nccih.nih.gov

NIH – National Center for Complementary and Integrative Health. "Meditation: In Depth." https://www.nccih.nih.gov

NHLBI- National Heart, Lung, and Blood Institute. "Study helps solve mystery of how sleep protects against heart disease." February 13, 2019. https://www.nhlbi.nih.gov

NIH- National Institute on Aging. "A Good Night's Sleep." https://www.nia.nih.gov

NSF- National Sleep Foundation. "National Sleep Foundation Recommends New Sleep Times." February 2, 2015. https://www.sleepfoundation.org

Nedergaard, Maiken, et al. "Sleep Drives Metabolite Clearance from the Adult Brain." October 2013. https://www.ncbi.nlm.nih.gov

Stewart, Jason, et al. "Maintaining the End: Roles of Telomere Proteins in End-Protection, Telomere Replication and Length Regulation." September 17, 2011. https://www.ncbi.nim.nih.gov

Vickers, Andrew, et al. "Acupuncture for Chronic Pain." October 22,2012. https://www.jamanetwork.com

WebMD. "Breathing Techniques for Stress Relief." January 7, 2018. https://www.webmd.com

White, A., Ernst, E. "A Brief History of Acupuncture." May 2004. https://www.academic.oup.com

CHAPTER 4—SPEND TIME IN NATURE

Alvarez, Sergio. "Health Check: why swimming in the sea is good for you." December 25, 2016. https://www.theconversation.com

CPSC -United States Consumer Product Safety Commission. "The Inside Story: A Guide to Indoor Air Quality." Accessed April 10, 2019. https://www.cpsc.gov

Dwyer-Lindgren, Laura, et al. "Inequalities in Life Expectancy Among US Counties, 1980 to 2014." July 2017. https://www.jamanetwork.com

EHP- Environmental Health Perspectives. "Exposure to Greenness and Mortality in a Nationwide Prospective Cohort Study of Women." September 1, 2016. https://www.ehp.niehs.nih.gov

Finlay, Jessica. "Therapeutic landscapes and wellbeing in later life: Impacts of blue and green spaces for older adults." May 2015. https://www.sciencedirect.com

Leary, Kyree. "China Will Plant 32,400 Square Miles of Trees to Combat Air Pollution." February 16, 2018. https://www.futurism.com

MedlinePlus. "Magnesium in diet." https://www.medlineplus.gov

National Center for Health Statistics. "Mortality in the United States, 2017." November 2018. https://www.cdc.com

Ong, Ling, Holland, Kim. "Bioerosion of coral reefs by two Hawaiian parrotfishes: species, size differences and fishery implications." June 2010. https://www.link.springer.com

Oschman, James, Chevalier, Gaetan, and Brown, Richard. "The effects of grounding (earthing) on inflammation, the immune response, wound healing, and prevention and treatment of chronic inflammatory and autoimmune diseases." March 24, 2015. https://www.ncbi.nim.nih.gov

Q, Li, et al. "Effect of phytoncide from trees on human natural killer cell function." October -December 2009. https://www.ncbi.nim.nih.gov

Raman, Ryan. "What Does Potassium Do for Your Body?" September 9, 2017. https://www.healthline.com

Science News. "Living at high altitude reduces risk of dying from heart disease: Low oxygen may spur genes to create blood vessels." March 26, 2011. https://www.sciencedaily.com

South, Eugenia, Hohl, Bernadette, Kondo, Michelle, et al. "Effect of Greening Vacant land on Mental Health of Community-Dwelling Adults." July 20, 2018. https://www.jamanetwork.com

Sukenik, S, et al. "Dead Sea bath salts for the treatment of rheumatoid arthritis." July-August 1990. https://www.ncbi.nim.nih.gov

WebMD. "Iodine." https://www.webmd.com

Yu, Chia-Pin, et al. "Effects of Short Forest Bathing Program on Autonomic Nervous System Activity and Mood

States in Middle-Aged and Elderly Individuals." August 9, 2017. https://www.ncbi.nlm.nih.gov

CHAPTER 5—TAKE CARE OF YOUR BRAIN

Adlaf, Elena, et al. "Adult-born neurons modify excitatory synaptic transmission to existing neurons." January 30, 2017. https://www.elifesciences.org

Alladi, Suvarna, Bak, Thomas, et al. "Bilingualism delays age at onset of dementia, independent of education and immigration status." November 26, 2013. https://www.n.neurology.org

Alzheimer's Association. https://www.alz.org

Baker, Kathi. "Musical activity may help the aging brain." April 22, 2011. https://www.emory.edu

Bavishi, A, et al. "A chapter a day: Association of book reading with longevity." July 18, 2016. https://www.ncbi.nim.nih.gov

Bever, Thomas, Chiarello, Robert. "Cerebral Dominance in Musicians and Nonmusicians." 2009. https://www.researchgate.net

Bolwerk, Anne, et al. "How Art Changes Your Brain: Differential Effects of Visual Art Production and Cognitive Art Evaluation on Functional Brain Connectivity." July 1, 2014. https://www.journals.plos.org

Bottiroli, Sara, et al. "The cognitive effects of listening to background music on older adults: processing speed improves with upbeat music, while memory seems to benefit from both upbeat and down beat music." October 15, 2014. https://www.frontiersin.org

Burgess, Lana. "12 foods to boost brain function." December 19, 2018. https://www.medicalnewstoday.com

Delistraty, Cody. "For a Better Brain, Learn Another Language." October 17, 2014. https://www.theatlantic.com

Forsythe, Paul, Bienenstock, John, Kunze, Wolfgang. "Vagal Pathways for Microbiome-Brain-Gut Axis Communication." June 9, 2014. https://www.springer.com

Huang, Rachel. "Scientists study music's effects on brain with fMRI." April 27, 2017. https://www.jhunewsletter.com

Kurtzman, Laura. "Training the Older Brain in 3-D: Video Game Enhances Cognitive Control." September 4, 2013. https://www.ucsf.edu

Langer, Ellen. 2009. *Counterclockwise: Mindful Health and the Power of Possibility*. New York. Ballantine Books. Quoted in Feinberg, Cara, "The Mindfulness Chronicles." Harvard Magazine. September-October 2010. https://www.harvardmagazine.com

Lapit, Amit, et al. "Computerized Cognitive Training in Cognitively Healthy Older Adults: A Systematic Review and Meta-Analysis of Effect Modifiers." November 18, 2014. https://www.journals.plos.org

Likova, Lora. "Drawing enhances cross-modal memory plasticity in the human brain: a case study in a totally blind adult." May 14, 2012. https://www.frontiersin.org

Marian, Viorica, et al. "Bilingual Cortical Control of Between-and Within- Language Competition." September 18, 2017. https://www.nature.com

Riedel, Brandalyn, et al. "Age, APOE and Sex: Triad of Risk of Alzheimer's Disease." March 8, 2016. https://www.ncbi.nim.nih.gov

Roberts, Rosebud, et al. "Risk and protective factors for cognitive impairment in persons aged 85 years and older." April 8, 2015. https://www.n.neurology.org Quoted in Tessman, Renee. "Can Arts, Crafts, and Computer Use Preserve Your Memory?" American Academy of Neurology. April 8, 2015.

Sylvia, Kristyn, Demas, Gregory. "A gut reaction: Microbiome-brain-immune interactions modulate social and affective behaviors." February 20, 2018. https://www.ncbi.nim.nih.gov

University of Sydney. "Does 'brain training' work?" November 18, 2014. https://www.eurekalert.org

Wan, Catherine and Schlaug, Gottfried. "Music Making as a Tool for Promoting Brain Plasticity across the Life Span." October 2010. https://www.ncbi.nlm.nih.gov

Wilson, Robert, et al. "Life-span cognitive activity, neuropathologic burden, and cognitive aging." July 3, 2013. https://www.n.neurology.org. Quoted in Song, Deb, "Does Being a Bookworm Boost Your Brainpower in Old Age?". Rush University Medical Center. 2013.

CHAPTER 6—ALLEVIATING TOXICITY

Alper, Lori. "Mom Detective: My Hunt for Non-Toxic Flooring." December 3, 2015. https://www.momscleanairforce.org

American Lung Association. "How can cleaning supplies, household product affect health?" https://www.lung.org

Anand, Preetha, et al. "Cancer is a Preventable Disease that Requires Major Lifestyle Changes." July 15, 2008. https://www.ncbi.nim.nih.gov

CPSC-United States Consumer Product Safety Commission. "The Inside Story: A Guide to Indoor Air Quality." https://www.cpsc.gov

EPA- Environmental Protection Agency. "Controlling Pollutants and Sources: Indoor Air Quality Design Tools for Schools." https://www.epa.gov

EPA–Environmental Protection Agency. "Volatile Organic Compounds' Impact on Indoor Air Quality." https://www.epa.gov

EWG- Environmental Working Group. "EWG's Healthy Living Home Guide." https://www.ewg.org

EWG – Environmental Working Group Staff. "Under New Safety Law, EPA Picks First 10 Chemicals For Review." December 7, 2016. https://www.ewg.org

FDA-U.S. Food & Drug Administration. "FDA in Brief: FDA issues final rule on safety and effectiveness for certain active ingredients in over-the-counter health care antiseptic hand washes and rubs in the medical setting." December 19, 2017. https://www.fda.gov

Imbeault, Pascal. "Can POPs be substantially popped out through sweat?" November 2017. https://www.sciencedirect.com

Jacobs, David, et al. "Carpets and Healthy Homes." https://www.nchh.org

The Lancet Commission. "The Lancet Commission on pollution and health." October 19,2017. https://www.thelancet.com

Narayan, Priyanka. "The cosmetics industry has avoided strict regulation for over a century. Now rising health concerns has FDA inquiring." August 2, 2018. https://www.cnbc.com

NIH-National Center for Complementary and Integrative Health. "Detoxes" and "Cleanses." https://www.nccih.nih.gov

NIH- National Heart, Lung, and Blood Institute. "How the Lungs Work." https://www.nhlbi.nih.gov

NIH- National Institute of Health. "Principles of Toxicology in the Context of Aging." 1987. https://www.ncbi. nim.nih.gov

Scialla,Mark. "It could take centuries for EPA to test all the unregulated chemicals under a new landmark bill." June 22, 2016. https://www.PBS.org

SciNews. "Scientists categorize Earth as a 'toxic planet.'" February 7, 2017. https://www.phys.org

Svanes, O, et al."Cleaning at Home and at Work in Relation to Lung Function Decline and Airway Obstruction." May 2018. https://www.ncbi.nlm.nih.gov

Thompson, Andrea. "The Truth about 'Green' Cleaning Products." August 6, 2007. https://www.livescience.com

West, Helen. "Himalayan Salt Lamps: Benefits and Myths." January 16, 2018. https://www.healthline.com

Winskowski, James. "This is Exactly Why Everybody Loves Salt Lamps." https://www.mindbodygreen.com

Wolverton, B.C. 1996. *How to Grow Fresh Air*. New York: Penguin Press.

WHO-World Health Organization. "9 out of 10 people worldwide breathe polluted air." May 2, 2018. https://www.who.int

Zerbe, Leah. "The 11 Safest Nontoxic Cleaners Plus What to Avoid)." September 10, 2012. https://www.prevention.com

CHAPTER 7—HAVE A PURPOSE IN LIFE

The Journals of Gerontology: Series A. "Does Private Religious Activity Prolong Survival? A Six-Year Follow-up Study of 3,851 Older Adults." July 1, 2000. https://www.academic.oup.com

Kim, Eric, et al. "Association Between Purpose in Life and Objective Measures of Physical Function in Older Adults." October 2007. https://www.jamanetwork.com

Koenig, Harold. "Religion, Spirituality, and Health: The Research and Clinical Implications." December 16,2012. https://www.ncbi.nim.nih.gov

Murthy, Vivek. "Work and the Loneliness Epidemic (Harvard Business Review)." September 27, 2017. https://www.vivekmurthy.com

Pew Research Center. "Where Americans Find Meaning in Life." November 20, 2018. https://www.pewforum.org

Salkin, Wendy. "Loneliness as epidemic." October 14, 2016. https://www.blog.petrieflom.law.harvard.edu

Turner, Arlene, et al. "Is Purpose in Life Associated with Less Sleep Disturbance in Older Adults?" July 10, 2017. https://www.sleep.biomedcentral.com

ACKNOWLEDGEMENTS

I would like to express my appreciation to my editor Deborah Ager for her insightful work on my manuscript. Her intelligence, thoroughness, and ability to bring clarity to my research was exactly what I needed.

My gratitude and love to my daughter, Heather Trimm, who functioned as my copy editor, website designer, and therapist when I faltered.

My deep appreciation to Dr. John Patton for setting me on the road to alternative health practices.

To Kevin Snow who opened my eyes to all the unseen wonders of this life.

I want to recognize the excellent work from Alise and Jeremy (Beehive Book Design). They produced a wonderful book cover design, a high-quality interior, and had endless patience with all the publishing questions from me, the novice author.

A thank you to Marti Statler, my marketing strategist, for her astute observations on how to attract readers for my book.

Finally, grateful thanks to my husband Mark and daughters, Heather and Tiffany, for all their support in both my journey with autoimmune disease and tolerance in listening to my never-ending discussions and angst over this book. It meant the world to me. Love you always.

Gretchen Adams is a writer and researcher living with autoimmune disease. In her past role as a media director for a national retail company, she worked in public speaking, research, print, radio, and television.

Gretchen and her husband spend winters in Florida and summers in the Rocky Mountains, which provides the perfect combination of weather and geography to inspire her watercolor and photography work.

If you are interested in learning more about how to live a healthier life, Gretchen can help. For more information about keynotes, workshops, and trainings, contact her at gretchenleeadams@gmail.com.

Bulk orders for your group are available at a discounted rate. Contact Gretchen directly for more information.

gretchenleeadams.com

Facebook.com/gretchenleeadams

Instagram.com/gretchenleeadams

Made in the
USA
Monee, IL